Current Topics in Canine and Feline Infectious Diseases

Guest Editor

STEPHEN C. BARR, BVSc, MVS, PhD

VETERINARY CLINICS OF NORTH AMERICA: SMALL ANIMAL PRACTICE

www.vetsmall.theclinics.com

November 2010 • Volume 40 • Number 6

SAUNDERS an imprint of ELSEVIER, Inc.

W.B. SAUNDERS COMPANY
A Division of Elsevier Inc.

1600 John F. Kennedy Blvd. ● Suite 1800 ● Philadelphia, PA 19103-2899
http://www.vetsmall.theclinics.com

**VETERINARY CLINICS OF NORTH AMERICA: SMALL ANIMAL PRACTICE Volume 40, Number 6
November 2010 ISSN 0195-5616, ISBN-13: 978-1-4377-2508-7**

Editor: John Vassallo; j.vassallo@elsevier.com
Developmental Editor: Jessica Demetriou

Veterinary Clinics of North America: Small Animal Practice (ISSN 0195-5616) is published bimonthly (For Post Office use only: volume 40 issue 6 of 6) by Elsevier Inc., 360 Park Avenue South, New York, NY 10010-1710. Months of issue are January, March, May, July, September, and November. Business and Editorial Offices: 1600 John F. Kennedy Blvd., Ste. 1800, Philadelphia, PA 19103-2899. Customer Service Office: 3251 Riverport Lane, Maryland Heights, MO 63043. Periodicals postage paid at New York, NY and additional mailing offices. Subscription prices are $262.00 per year (domestic individuals), $427.00 per year (domestic institutions), $128.00 per year (domestic students/residents), $347.00 per year (Canadian individuals), $525.00 per year (Canadian institutions), $385.00 per year (international individuals), $525.00 per year (international institutions), and $186.00 per year (international and Canadian students/residents). To receive student/resident rate, orders must be accompanied by name of affiliated institution, date of term, and the *signature* of program/residency coordinator on institution letterhead. Orders will be billed at individual rate until proof of status is received. Foreign air speed delivery is included in all *Clinics* subscription prices. All prices are subject to change without notice. **POSTMASTER:** Send address changes to *Veterinary Clinics of North America: Small Animal Practice*, Elsevier Health Sciences Division, Subscription Customer Service, 3251 Riverport Lane, Maryland Heights, MO 63043. Customer Service (orders, claims, online, change of address): Elsevier Periodicals Customer Service, Elsevier Health Sciences Division Subscription Customer Service 3251 Riverport Lane Maryland Heights, MO 63043. Tel: 1-800-654-2452 (U.S. and Canada); 314-447-8871 (outside U.S. and Canada). Fax: 314-447-8029. E-mail: journalscustomerservice-usa@elsevier.com (for print support); journalsonlinesupport-usa@elsevier.com (for online support).

Reprints. For copies of 100 or more of articles in this publication, please contact the Commercial Reprints Department, Elsevier Inc., 360 Park Avenue South, New York, NY 10010-1710. Tel.: 212-633-3812; Fax: 212-462-1935; E-mail: reprints@elsevier.com.

Veterinary Clinics of North America: Small Animal Practice is also published in Japanese by Inter Zoo Publishing Co., Ltd., Aoyama Crystal-Bldg 5F, 3-5-12 Kitaaoyama, Minato-ku, Tokyo 107-0061, Japan.

Veterinary Clinics of North America: Small Animal Practice is covered in *Current Contents/Agriculture, Biology and Environmental Sciences, Science Citation Index, ASCA, MEDLINE/PubMed (Index Medicus), Excerpta Medica, and BIOSIS.*

Printed in the United States of America.

Contributors

GUEST EDITOR

STEPHEN C. BARR, BVSc, MVS, PhD
Diplomate, American College of Veterinary Internal Medicine; Professor of Medicine, Department of Clinical Sciences, College of Veterinary Medicine, Cornell University, Ithaca, New York

AUTHORS

EDWARD J. DUBOVI, PhD
Diplomate, American College of Veterinary Microbiologists; Professor and Director of Virology, Department of Population and Diagnostic Sciences, Animal Health Diagnostic Center, College of Veterinary Medicine, Cornell University, Ithaca, New York

DANIEL S. FOY, MS, DVM
Diplomate, American College of Veterinary Internal Medicine; Emergency and Critical Care Fellow, Department of Medical Sciences, School of Veterinary Medicine, University of Wisconsin-Madison, Madison, Wisconsin

AMELIA GODDARD, BVSc, MMedVet
Associate Professor of Clinical Pathology, Department of Companion Animal Clinical Studies, Faculty of Veterinary Science, University of Pretoria, Onderstepoort, Pretoria, South Africa

RICHARD E. GOLDSTEIN, DVM
Diplomate, European College of Veterinary Internal Medicine - Companion Animals; Diplomate, American College of Veterinary Internal Medicine; Associate Professor of Medicine, Department of Clinical Sciences, College of Veterinary Medicine, Cornell University, Ithaca, New York

LYNN GUPTILL, DVM, PhD
Diplomate, American College of Veterinary Internal Medicine; Associate Professor of Small Animal Internal Medicine, Department of Veterinary Clinical Sciences, Purdue University, West Lafayette, Indiana

PETER J. IRWIN, BVetMed, PhD, FACVSc, MRCVS
Associate Professor of Small Animal Medicine, Department of Veterinary Clinical Science, School of Veterinary and Biomedical Sciences, Murdoch University, Murdoch, Western Australia, Australia

INKE KRUPKA, Dr Med Vet
Chair for Bacteriology and Mycology, Institute for Infectious Diseases and Zoonoses, Department of Veterinary Sciences, Ludwig-Maximilians-University, Munich, Germany

MICHAEL R. LAPPIN, DVM, PhD
Diplomate, American College of Veterinary Internal Medicine; Professor, Department of Clinical Sciences, Colorado State University, Fort Collins, Colorado

ANDREW L. LEISEWITZ, BVSc, MMedVet, PhD
Professor of Medicine, Department of Companion Animal Clinical Studies, Faculty of Veterinary Science, University of Pretoria, Onderstepoort, Pretoria, South Africa

SUSAN E. LITTLE, DVM, PhD
Diplomate, European Veterinary Parasitology College; Professor and Krull-Ewing Chair in Veterinary Parasitology, Center for Veterinary Health Sciences, Oklahoma State University, Stillwater, Oklahoma

DAVID J. MAGGS, BVSc (Hons)
Diplomate, American College of Veterinary Ophthalmologists; Associate Professor, Department of Surgical and Radiological Sciences, School of Veterinary Medicine, University of California, Davis, California

REINHARD K. STRAUBINGER, PhD
Professor, Chair for Bacteriology and Mycology, Institute for Infectious Diseases and Zoonoses, Department of Veterinary Sciences, Ludwig-Maximilians-University, Munich, Germany

JANE E. SYKES, BVSc(Hon), PhD
Diplomate, American College of Veterinary Internal Medicine; Professor, Department of Medicine and Epidemiology, University of California Davis, Davis, California

LAUREN A. TREPANIER, DVM, PhD
Diplomate, American College of Veterinary Internal Medicine; Diplomate, American College of Veterinary Clinical Pharmacology; Professor, Department of Medical Sciences, School of Veterinary Medicine, University of Wisconsin-Madison, Madison, Wisconsin

JULIA K. VEIR, DVM, PhD
Diplomate, American College of Veterinary Internal Medicine; Assistant Professor, Department of Clinical Sciences, Colorado State University, Fort Collins, Colorado

Contents

> Since its emergence in 1978, canine parvoviral enteritis has remained a common and important cause of morbidity and mortality in young dogs. The continued incidence of parvoviral enteritis is partly due to the virus's capability to "reinvent" itself and evolve into new, more virulent and resistant subspecies. This article reviews current knowledge about the virus, its epidemiology, clinical manifestation, diagnosis, management, and prevention.

> A large variety of antiviral agents exists for oral or topical treatment of cats infected with feline herpesvirus type 1. Knowledge of the general principles can be used to better understand antiviral pharmacology and thereby guide therapy for cats with herpetic disease. This article compares the antiviral efficacy of these compounds and recommends a common protocol for administering lysine and antiviral drugs to infected cats.

> Canine influenza, as a recognized clinical entity in dogs, has a relatively brief history. The presence of specific subtypes of influenza virus capable of being transmitted from dog to dog is at present geographically limited to the United States and Korea. As surveillance intensifies to meet the concerns of the human population on pandemic influenza viruses, more cases of influenza virus in dogs are certain to be detected. Each infection offers an opportunity for a unique variant to emerge and continue the evolution of influenza virus as a species-crossing pathogen.

> *Bartonella* infection is common among domestic cats, but the role of *Bartonella* species as feline pathogens requires further study. Most *Bartonella* species that infect cats are zoonotic. Cats are the mammalian reservoir and vector for *Bartonella henselae*, an important zoonotic agent. Cat fleas transmit *Bartonella* among cats, and cats with fleas are an important source of human *B henselae* infections. New information about *Bartonella* as feline pathogens has recently been published, and this article summarizes much of that information. Issues surrounding diagnosis and treatment of feline *Bartonella* infections are described, and prevention of zoonotic transmission of *Bartonella* is discussed.

> Leptospirosis is a common zoonotic disease with a worldwide distribution. Dogs become infected by exposure to contaminated urine from shedding wild animals. The bacteria penetrate mucus membranes, causing endothelial damage and damage to organs, such as the liver and kidneys. The clinical signs and clinicopathologic data are nonspecific and a high index of suspicion is needed by the practitioner. Testing today is highly based on serology (microscopic agglutination test) and perhaps polymerase chain reaction. Treatment of leptospirosis involves supportive care and antibiotics, and prevention includes environmental steps and annual vaccination of dogs at risk.

> Lyme borreliosis (LB), synonymous with the often-used term Lyme disease, is an infectious disease caused by the spirochetal bacterium *Borrelia burgdorferi*. LB is the most frequent vector-borne disease in humans in the Northern Hemisphere. In animals, clinically apparent disease is found primarily in dogs. Severe polyarthritis, fever and lameness in dogs are reported from the main endemic areas of North America: the New England States, and eastern parts of the United States; several cases of LB are also seen in California and the Midwest. Because of the difficulties in finding sufficient indicative clinical signs, additional information (detailed case history, laboratory testing for antibodies) is especially important to make the clinical diagnosis of Lyme borreliosis. This article reviews the etiology, diagnosis, therapy, and prevention of LB.

> In the time since canine ehrlichiosis due to *Ehrlichia canis* was first described in 1935 and first recognized in the United States in 1962, many key advances have been made in our understanding of the diversity of the rickettsial organisms responsible for ehrlichiosis and anaplasmosis in dogs and, occasionally, cats, the vectors capable of transmitting these agents, and the role these organisms play as both important veterinary pathogens and zoonotic disease agents. Despite considerable progress in the field, much remains to be learned regarding mechanisms contributing to pathogenesis, effective treatment modalities, and prevention strategies that best protect pet health. This article highlights current understanding of the transmission, diagnosis, and management of ehrlichiosis and anaplasmosis in dogs and cats.

> Babesiosis continues to pose a threat to dogs worldwide as a cause of anemia, thrombocytopenia, and a wide variety of clinical signs, ranging from mild, nonspecific illness to peracute collapse and death. Practitioners

should be alert to the importance of collecting travel and fight history for a patient and should be aware of new piroplasm species that have been described. Asymptomatic infections necessitate careful screening of potential blood donors using a combination of diagnostic testing procedures. Current treatment strategies for babesiosis often ameliorate the clinical signs of infection, but these hemoparasites are seldom completely eliminated, and when immunocompromised, recrudescence may occur.

Three species of hemotropic mycoplasmas are known to infect cats worldwide, *Mycoplasma haemofelis,* "*Candidatus* Mycoplasma turicensis" and "*Candidatus* Mycoplasma haemominutum." These organisms were previously known as *Haemobartonella felis*, but are now known to be mycoplasmas. Assays based on polymerase chain reaction technology are the most sensitive and specific diagnostic tests available for these organisms. *M haemofelis* is the most pathogenic species, and causes hemolytic anemia in immunocompetent cats. Other differential diagnoses for hemolytic anemia should be considered in cats testing positive for "*Candidatus* Mycoplasma turicensis" and "*Candidatus* Mycoplasma haemominutum," because the presence of these organisms is not always associated with anemia. Blood from infected cats should be handled with care because of the potential zoonotic nature of hemoplasma infections. The treatment of choice for cats with clinical disease is doxycycline.

Antifungal therapy has progressed significantly with the development of new drugs directed at various processes in fungal cell metabolism. Within veterinary medicine, treatment options for systemic mycoses remain limited to amphotericin B, ketoconazole, fluconazole, and itraconazole. However, newer triazoles, echinocandins, and lipid-based formulations of amphotericin B are now approved for use in humans. This article provides a comprehensive review of the antifungal medications available for veterinary patients, and includes a brief discussion of the newer, presently cost-prohibitive, antifungal therapies used for systemic mycoses in humans.

With the advent of more accessible polymerase chain reaction panels, the use of molecular techniques for the detection of infectious organisms has become more routine in veterinary medicine. The use of molecular diagnostics is best reserved for the detection of organisms that are difficult to detect or identify expediently. In this article, the fundamentals of molecular techniques are reviewed along with an examination of specific feline infectious diseases in which diagnosis via molecular techniques is advantageous.

FORTHCOMING ISSUES

January 2011
Kidney Failure and Renal Replacement Therapies
Mark Acierno, MBA, DVM and
Mary A. Labato, DVM, *Guest Editors*

March 2011
Organ Failure in Critical Illness
Tim Hackett, DVM, MS,
Guest Editor

May 2011
Chronic Intestinal Diseases of Dogs and Cats
Frédéric Gaschen, Dr Med Vet, Dr Habil,
Guest Editor

RECENT ISSUES

September 2010
Spinal Diseases
Ronaldo C. da Costa, DMV, MSc, PhD,
Guest Editor

July 2010
Topics in Cardiology
Jonathan A. Abbott, DVM,
Guest Editor

May 2010
Immunology: Function, Pathology, Diagnostics, and Modulation
Melissa A. Kennedy, DVM, PhD,
Guest Editor

RELATED INTEREST

Veterinary Clinics of North America: Exotic Animal Practice
September 2009 (Vol. 12, No. 3)
Bacterial and Parasitic Diseases
Laura Wade, DVM, Dipl. ABVP—Avian, *Guest Editor*

THE CLINICS ARE NOW AVAILABLE ONLINE!

Access your subscription at:
www.theclinics.com

Preface

Current Topics in Canine and Feline Infectious Diseases

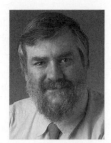

Stephen C. Barr, BVSc, MVS, PhD
Guest Editor

I thank the editorial staff of Elsevier for the opportunity to bring together current glimpses into several infectious diseases which are important to the veterinary practitioner. The experts I approached are all active veterinary scientists doing outstanding research on their chosen infectious disease. This is not to say there are no others working on these diseases, but these authors, I believe, have moved the science forward significantly. Not all authors are living and working in America; it is important to realize the outstanding knowledge contributed by our colleagues overseas. Some primary authors are just starting out in their careers; it is essential we encourage and feed our junior colleagues as they will provide the creativity behind continued advances in the future.

Each author was asked to write a review emphasizing the biology and current diagnostic and treatment strategies for these diseases that would help practicing veterinarians in their everyday trade. Some topics, such as parvovirus, leptospirosis, borreliosis, babesiosis, and hemotrophic mycoplasmas, would seemingly be old hat. However, I think the authors of these articles have provided new insights into these diseases. One topic (canine influenza) is truly a new disease and needs careful attention by practicing veterinarians. Others, such as herpes viruses and feline bartonellosis, have been around for a good while but are receiving new attention. The article on ehrlichiosis also puts this topic in perspective for the practitioner.

Of particular interest to practitioners, I think, will be the topic of molecular diagnostics for feline infectious diseases. Molecular diagnostic techniques can be very useful but, as this article points out, the results have to be carefully assessed based on knowledge of the particular pitfalls of the test; in other words, as with all diagnostic tests, the practicing veterinarian needs to consider very carefully the consequences of a positive and negative result for that particular pet.

Vet Clin Small Anim 40 (2010) ix–x
doi:10.1016/j.cvsm.2010.07.013
0195-5616/10/$ – see front matter © 2010 Elsevier Inc. All rights reserved.

vetsmall.theclinics.com

I have learned much from these authors as this issue has taken shape. For that, I thank them, but I especially thank them for their tireless scientific rigor in moving veterinary medicine forward as a science and away from a voodoo art form. It is only through the practice of science and not religion, hunches, or hearsay will veterinary medicine truly progress.

Stephen C. Barr, BVSc, MVS, PhD
Vet Box 32
College of Veterinary Medicine
Cornell University
Ithaca, NY 14853, USA

E-mail address:
scb6@cornell.edu

Canine Parvovirus

Amelia Goddard, BVSc, MMedVet*,
Andrew L. Leisewitz, BVSc, MMedVet, PhD

KEYWORDS

• Parvovirus • Canine • Hemorrhagic enteritis • Vaccination

Since its emergence in 1978, canine parvoviral enteritis was and remains a common and important cause of morbidity and mortality in young dogs. The continued incidence of parvoviral enteritis is partly due to the virus's capability to "reinvent" itself and evolve into new more virulent and resistant subspecies. Here the authors review current knowledge about the virus, its epidemiology, clinical manifestation, diagnosis, management, and prevention.

PARVOVIRIDAE

Parvoviruses (Parvoviridae) are small, nonenveloped, single-stranded DNA viruses that are known to cause disease in a variety of mammalian species, although most parvoviruses are species specific.[1–3] Parvovirus requires the host cell for replication, specifically the cell nucleus, and binds the host cell by the double-stranded ends of the genome. Viral replication occurs only in rapidly dividing cells such as intestinal crypt epithelial cells, precursor cells in the bone marrow, and myocardiocytes. Viral replication results in cell death and loss due to failure of mitosis.[2–4] Not all rapidly dividing cell populations are equally affected, suggesting a viral tropism for certain target organs.[4]

EPIDEMIOLOGY

The virus is better known as canine parvovirus type 2 (CPV-2) because it was the second parvovirus described in dogs. In 1967, parvovirus was first discovered as a cause of gastrointestinal and respiratory disease in dogs, and was then called the minute virus of canines.[5] It was later designated CPV-1. Most patients infected with CPV-1 are asymptomatic.[3] In 1978, reports of outbreaks of an unfamiliar contagious enteric disease were reported in the United States. The causal agent was isolated and data showed that it was a new species of the genus Parvoviridae; it was subsequently named CPV-2. Due to the lack of preexisting immunity in the canine population, the virus spread rapidly and by 1980 it was reported to be common worldwide.[1,3]

Department of Companion Animal Clinical Studies, Faculty of Veterinary Science, University of Pretoria, Private Bag X04, Onderstepoort, Pretoria 0110, South Africa
* Corresponding author.
E-mail address: amelia.goddard@up.ac.za

Vet Clin Small Anim 40 (2010) 1041–1053
doi:10.1016/j.cvsm.2010.07.007
0195-5616/10/$ – see front matter © 2010 Elsevier Inc. All rights reserved.

The exact origin and evolution of CPV-2 is still a debated issue. Some reports found it to be closely related to feline panleukopenia virus and several publications did suggest that CPV-2 may have originated from this virus.[4] Other research suggests that CPV-2 originated from an antigenically similar ancestor, such as a wild carnivore.[3,6] Initially the infection led to high morbidity and mortality in the naïve canine population, but after the introduction of vaccines, outbreaks were limited to unvaccinated or improperly vaccinated animals and shelter environments. In the 1980s a new CPV-2 strain emerged and was designated CPV-2a. The virus quickly mutated again and a new strain, CPV-2b, emerged in 1984.[3,7] Today, CPV-2a and CPV-2b are still the most common parvovirus species causing disease in canines globally. Within the past decade a new strain, CPV-2c, has emerged. This strain was first reported in Italy in 2000[8] and was soon also reported in Vietnam,[9] Spain,[10] the United States,[11] South America,[12] Portugal,[13] Germany, and the United Kingdom.[14] This strain is claimed to be highly virulent, with high morbidity and rapid death.

Acute CPV-2 enteritis can be seen in dogs of any breed, age, or sex, but puppies between 6 weeks and 6 months of age appear to be more susceptible.[6,15,16] Immunity to CPV following infection or vaccination is long lived, and therefore the only susceptible pool of animals is puppies born into the population. For the first few weeks of life puppies are protected against infection by maternally derived antibody (assuming the bitch has antibodies). Disease is therefore seldom encountered in neonates.[17] However, maternal antibody to parvovirus has a half-life of approximately 10 days, and as their maternal antibody titers decline puppies become susceptible to infection.[17,18]

Factors that predispose to parvoviral infection in puppies are lack of protective immunity, intestinal parasites, and overcrowded, unsanitary, and stressful environmental conditions.[2,15,19] Certain breeds have been shown to be at increased risk for severe CPV enteritis, including the rottweiler, doberman pinscher, American pit bull terrier, Labrador retriever, and German shepherd dog.[2,19,20] Reasons for breed susceptibility are unclear. Common ancestry in the doberman pinscher and rottweiler, the fact that both breeds have a relatively higher prevalence of von Willebrand's disease (VWD), as well as inherited immunodeficiency in rottweilers have been implicated.[16,20,21] Besides a genetic component, other factors may also account for increased risk of disease, such as breed popularity and lack of appropriate vaccination protocols.[16] Among dogs older than 6 months, sexually intact males appear to be twice as likely to develop CPV enteritis as sexually intact females.[20] A distinct seasonality has also been reported, with peak incidence of disease during summer months and a trough during winter.[20,22]

PATHOGENESIS

CPV-2 spreads rapidly among dogs via the fecal-oral route (direct transmission) or through oronasal exposure to fomites contaminated by feces (indirect transmission).[2,15,23] Fecal excretion of the virus has been shown to be as early as 3 days after experimental inoculation, and shedding may continue for a maximum period of 3 to 4 weeks after clinical or subclinical disease.[23,24] Virus replication begins in the lymphoid tissue of the oropharynx, mesenteric lymph nodes, and thymus, and is disseminated to the intestinal crypts of the small intestine by hematogenous spread (3–4 days after infection).[2,6,15,25,26] Marked plasma viremia is observed 1 to 5 days after infection. Subsequent to the viremia, CPV-2 localizes predominantly in the epithelium lining the tongue, oral cavity, and esophagus; the small intestine; bone marrow; and lymphoid tissue, such as thymus and lymph nodes.[15,24,26,27] Virus has been isolated from lungs, spleen, liver, kidneys, and myocardium, showing that CPV infection is a systemic disease.[2,15,25]

The rate of lymphoid and intestinal cell turnover appears to be the main factor determining the severity of the disease: higher rates of turnover are directly correlated with virus replication and cell destruction. Stress factors, in particular parasitic and nonspecific factors (eg, weaning), may predispose dogs to clinical disease by increasing mucosal cell activity.[2,6,23,28,29] During weaning, enterocytes of the intestinal crypts have a higher mitotic index because of the changes in bacterial flora and diet, and are therefore more susceptible to the viral tropism for rapidly dividing cells.[20]

Intestinal crypt epithelial cells maturing in the small intestine normally migrate from the germinal epithelium of the crypts to the tips of the villi. On reaching the villous tips, they acquire their absorptive capability and aid in assimilating nutrients. Parvovirus infects the germinal epithelium of the intestinal crypt, causing epithelial destruction and villous collapse. As a result, normal cell turnover (usually 1–3 days in the small intestine) is impaired, leading to the characteristic pathologic lesion of shortened and atrophic villi.[2,6,15,30,31] During this period of villous atrophy the small intestine loses its absorptive capacity. The changes in the thymus are dramatic. The lesions are usually most obvious in the germinal centers and the thymic cortex, reflecting the tropism of CPV for mitotically active cell populations. The extensive lymphocytolysis in the thymic cortex, as compared with other lymphoid tissues, further reflects the high mitotic rate found in this organ, and it is thus not surprising that infected puppies develop severe lymphopenia.[2,32]

CLINICAL MANIFESTATION

Enteritis and myocarditis were the 2 disease entities initially described with CPV-2 infection. CPV-2 myocarditis is very rarely seen nowadays, but can develop from infection in utero or in puppies less than 8 weeks old born to unvaccinated bitches.[15] In this scenario usually all puppies in a litter are affected, often being found dead or succumbing within 24 hours after the appearance of clinical signs. The onset and progression of clinical disease is rapid, and clinical signs include dyspnea, crying, and retching.[15,33] The myocardial lesion is multifocal necrosis and lysis of myofibers with or without an inflammatory response. Intranuclear inclusion bodies can be found within the myocardial cell nuclei.[34]

Acute enteritis is the most common manifestation of the disease and is mostly seen in puppies up to 6 months of age. Initial clinical signs are nonspecific, and include anorexia, depression, lethargy, and fever. Later typical signs include vomiting and small bowel diarrhea that can range from mucoid to hemorrhagic.[3,16] Due to large fluid and protein losses through the gastrointestinal tract, dehydration and hypovolemic shock often develop rapidly.[16] Marked abdominal pain is often a feature of CPV enteritis and can be caused by either acute gastroenteritis or intestinal intussusception.

Intestinal tract damage secondary to viral infection increases the risk of bacterial translocation and subsequent coliform septicemia, which may lead to the development of a systemic inflammatory response that can progress to septic shock and, ultimately, death. *Escherichia coli* has been recovered from the lungs and liver of infected puppies. Pulmonary lesions similar to those found in humans with adult respiratory distress syndrome have been described.[16,31,35] It has also been suggested that the hemorrhagic diarrhea is a consequence of endotoxemia and cytokine production and does not derive directly from viral infection.[36] Research data have shown that endotoxin and tumor necrosis factor (TNF) are present in measurable quantities in the blood of infected puppies and that a significant association exists between rising TNF activity and mortality.[31] Endotoxin and proinflammatory cytokines are potent mediators of the systemic inflammatory response and activators of the coagulation cascade.[37,38]

No specific radiographic signs are associated with CPV enteritis besides those typically seen in gastroenteritis, that is, fluid- and gas-filled bowel loops. A recent study has examined the ultrasonographic appearance of CPV enteritis in comparison with that of normal puppies.[39,40] Although none of the ultrasonographic changes were pathognomonic for CPV enteritis, the combination of changes was highly suggestive of the disease. Typical changes that were considered indicative of CPV enteritis included fluid-filled, atonic small and large intestines; duodenal and jejunal mucosal layer thinning with or without indistinct wall layers and irregular luminal-mucosal surfaces; extensive duodenal and/or jejunal hyperechoic mucosal speckling; and duodenal and/or jejunal corrugations. The extensive intestinal lesions correlated with the histopathological findings of villous sloughing, mucosal erosion and ulceration, and crypt necrosis. In this study CPV infection did not appear to be associated with sonographically detectable lymphadenopathy. The severity of the sonographic changes did correlate with the clinical condition of the patients.[39,40]

CLINICOPATHOLOGIC FEATURES

The leukocyte count during CPV enteritis is generally characterized as significantly depressed, with a transient lymphopenia being the most consistent finding. The hematological changes are widely accepted to be attributable to destruction of hematopoietic progenitor cells of the various leukocyte types in the bone marrow and other lymphoproliferative organs such as the thymus, lymph nodes, and spleen. This process results in inadequate supply for the massive demand for leukocytes (specifically neutrophils) in the inflamed gastrointestinal tract.[32,41] A recent study showed that a lack of cytopenia, specifically the total leukocyte and lymphocyte counts, had a positive predictive value of 100% for survival 24 hours post admission. A rebound increase in the lymphocyte count 24 hours after admission was seen in the puppies that recovered.[41] Studies have also shown a marked depletion of the granulocytic, erythroid, and megakaryocytic cell lines in the bone marrow followed by hyperplasia of the granulocytic and erythroid elements during convalescence.[42,43] These changes are nonspecific and could reflect the effect of endotoxemia.[43] Despite the severe changes seen in the blood precursor cell lines, it appears that early pluripotent cells are spared.[32] Increased plasma granulocyte colony-stimulating factor (G-CSF) concentration has been observed in CPV enteritis just after the onset of neutropenia, which then decreases to undetectable levels once the neutropenia has resolved.[44]

Anemia is not an uncommon hematological finding in CPV enteritis, especially in the later phases of severe disease. The cause of this is unlikely to be suppression of erythropoiesis, as circulating red blood cells have a long half-life relative to the short period during which the virus suppresses production in the bone marrow.[42] Reduced hematocrit is more likely to be the result of a combination of intestinal hemorrhage and rehydration therapy.[15,28] Increased levels of lipid peroxides and an alteration in antioxidant enzyme concentrations, indicating a state of oxidative stress in these patients, may also play a role in anemia pathogenesis.[45]

Virus-induced thrombocytopenia can occur because of decreased platelet production or as a result of direct action of viruses and/or immunologic components on platelets or endothelium.[46] Besides hemorrhagic manifestations (which are rare), subclinical thrombocytopenia may affect vascular permeability, which may potentiate extravascular dissemination of the virus.[47] Evidence of hypercoagulability without disseminated intravascular coagulopathy has been documented in puppies with CPV enteritis and is thought to be due to an endotoxin- or cytokine-mediated procoagulant effect on endothelial cells. Loss of antithrombin (AT) through the gastrointestinal tract, as well as consumption of AT as a result of endotoxin-mediated activation of coagulation, and hyperfibrinogenemia are thought to contribute to the hypercoagulable state seen in CPV enteritis.[48]

The response of the adrenal and thyroid glands to critical illness is essential for survival. Similar to critical illness in humans, high serum cortisol and low serum thyroxine (T4) concentrations at 24 and 48 hours after admission are associated with death in puppies with CPV enteritis.[49,50]

Infection-induced serum chemistry abnormalities are nonspecific. Severe hypokalemia due to anorexia, vomiting, and diarrhea may contribute to depression and weakness. Other electrolyte abnormalities (ie, hyponatremia and hypochloremia) may also occur secondary to vomiting and diarrhea.[28,51,52] Although total magnesium concentration has been found to be a prognostic indicator in critically ill humans, total as well as ionized magnesium concentrations were not associated with outcome in CPV enteritis.[53] Hypoalbuminemia may contribute to reduced total blood calcium concentrations.[28] Serum electrophoresis profiles have shown relative and absolute hypoalbuminemia, hypogammaglobulinemia, and hyper–α2-globulinemia.[54] The decrease in plasma proteins through the course of the disease are mostly due to a combination of intestinal hemorrhage followed by rehydration. The increase in α2-globulins are most likely due to the hepatic synthesis of acute phase proteins (APP) stimulated by leukocyte endogenous mediators that are associated with tissue damage and inflammation.[54] Acute-phase protein generation occurs at the expense of albumin generation in critical illness.[55] Unpublished data on serum C-reactive protein (CRP), a major APP in the dog, have shown that higher CRP levels at admission, and 12 and 24 hours after admission are positively associated with an increased risk of mortality (unpublished data from McClure V and colleagues, Faculty of Veterinary Science, University of Pretoria, South Africa, 2010). Elevated blood urea, creatinine, and inorganic phosphate are associated with dehydration. Elevation in alkaline phosphatase and alanine transaminase may occur as a result of hepatic hypoxia secondary to severe hypovolemia or the absorption of toxic substances due to loss of the gut barrier. Elevated alkaline phosphatase activity can also be associated with young age.[28,51] Plasma lipoproteins bind the bioactive portion of the endotoxin (LPS) molecule, preventing it from stimulating monocytes, macrophages, and other LPS-responsive cells thereby providing an important host mechanism for controlling responses to endotoxin. Several reports have shown a strong correlation between low plasma cholesterol and mortality in critically ill and infected human patients. A recent study has shown serum total cholesterol and high-density lipoprotein cholesterol levels to decrease, but serum triglyceride levels to increase in CPV enteritis. Hypocholesterolemia may be used as an index of the severity of CPV enteritis.[56]

Studies on acid-base status in CPV enteritis have shown puppies to develop either acidosis or alkalosis depending on the severity of the vomiting (ie, loss of hydrogen and chloride ions) or the origin of the diarrhea (ie, small versus large intestine).[52] The majority of cases show a decrease in venous blood pH and HCO_3^-, which indicate the development of metabolic acidosis probably caused by excessive loss of HCO_3^- through the intestinal tract.[57,58] The metabolic acidosis seen in CPV enteritis is, however, readily corrected and is not exacerbated by D-lactate production by the bacterial population within the large intestine.[58]

DIAGNOSIS

Despite the typical presentation seen with CPV infection of acute-onset vomiting and diarrhea, depression, dehydration, fever, and leukopenia in an unvaccinated puppy, these findings are nonspecific although this cluster of findings is frequently the legitimate basis of a presumptive diagnosis. Definitive diagnostic tests include demonstration of CPV in the feces of affected dogs, serology, and necropsy with histopathology.[59] Diagnosis of active CPV infection via serology requires detection of anti-CPV antibody that is of recent origin (ie, IgM class antibodies) in the face of typical clinical signs.[60] A near-patient enzyme-linked immunosorbent assay test is available to practitioners to demonstrate CPV in the feces of infected puppies.[61] Viral particles are readily detectable at the peak of shedding (4–7 days after infection).[59] False-positive results may occur 3 to 10 days post vaccination with a modified live CPV vaccine, and false-negative results may occur secondary to binding of serum-neutralizing antibodies with antigen in diarrhea or cessation of fecal viral shed.[6,16,51] Other methods available to detect CPV antigen in feces include electron microscopy, viral isolation, fecal hemagglutination, latex agglutination, counterimmunoelectrophoresis, immunochromatography, and polymerase chain reaction (PCR).[51,59,62,63] PCR-based methods, specifically real-time PCR, have been shown to be more sensitive than traditional techniques.[62]

MANAGEMENT

Canine parvoviral enteritis is associated with a survival rate as low as 9.1% in the absence of treatment, and 64% or higher with treatment.[31] Because no agent-specific treatment exists for CPV enteritis, management of this condition remains supportive care. Mildly affected puppies may be treated on an outpatient basis. Outpatient treatment cannot, however, be recommended, because most of these puppies will deteriorate as owners frequently fail to maintain oral treatment programs in the face of worsening vomiting. Best management requires admission and aggressive treatment with crystalloid fluids, synthetic and natural colloids, correction of hypoglycemia and any electrolyte disturbances, combination antimicrobials, antiemetics, analgesics, enteral nutritional support, and anthelmintics. Fluid therapy to treat dehydration, reestablish effective circulating blood volume, as well as correct electrolyte and acid-base disturbances is the mainstay of managing more severely affected puppies.[16,51] Fluid therapy in these patients can be complex, and careful attention should be paid to physical examination in addition to electrolyte and acid-base status.[64] The preferred route of administration is intravenous, but intraosseus administration, although rarely used, may be useful in patients that need rapid fluid administration when intravenous access is impossible. It is crucial that all intravenous catheterization procedures be aseptic and catheter care be fastidious, as catheter-induced infection (abscessation and cellulites that may extend to septic polyarthritis and discospondylitis) is a serious complication in these immunosuppressed puppies. All intravenous catheters should be replaced after 72 hours of use.[65] Isotonic crystalloid solutions can be administered either subcutaneously or intraperitoneally to treat mild dehydration, but this is contraindicated in the face of circulatory compromise because of inadequate distribution secondary to peripheral vasoconstriction, as well as the risk of infection in severely leukopenic patients.[16,64] The initial fluid of choice is a balanced electrolyte solution that is isotonic to blood (ie, lactated Ringer solution). The initial rate of fluid administration will depend on the condition of the patient. Fluid deficits should be replaced as soon as possible (within 1–6 hours of presentation).[16,51] Once perfusion is restored the intravenous fluid rate is reduced to a maintenance rate plus estimated ongoing losses. Puppies with CPV enteritis are prone to develop hypokalemia and hypoglycemia (specifically toy breeds) due to ongoing anorexia, vomiting, and diarrhea. Severe hypokalemia can result in profound muscle weakness, gastrointestinal ileus, cardiac arrhythmias, and polyuria.[16,51] Both serum potassium and glucose, together with the packed cell volume (PCV) and total serum protein, should be monitored at least once a day. Potassium chloride should be added to the fluids according to the patient's requirements. The amount of potassium chloride administered should be calculated and the clinician should ensure that the rate does not exceed 0.5 mEq/kg/h, as it may have adverse effects on normal cardiac function.[64] Supplementation of dextrose added to the balanced electrolyte solution to a final concentration of 2.5% to 5% may be necessary to prevent hypoglycemia once the initial critical hypoglycemia has been addressed.[16,51]

Puppies suffering from CPV enteritis often develop a severe protein-losing enteropathy due to the destruction of intestinal villi, and therefore the addition of a nonprotein colloid (ie, hetastarch or dextran 70) should be considered when total protein drops below 35 g/L (albumin <20 g/L) or if the patient shows evidence of loss of fluid into a third space.[16,51] Overzealous colloidal therapy must be avoided to prevent blunting of endogenous hepatic albumin production.[16,55] The role of blood products in the treatment of CPV is controversial. Patients suffering from anemia secondary to hemorrhagic diarrhea or concurrent endoparasitism, and showing clinical signs referable to anemia, can be treated with packed red blood cells or whole blood. Fresh frozen plasma (FFP) transfusion has been recommended in the treatment of CPV enteritis for its ability to provide oncotic components (albumin), immunoglobulins, and serum protease inhibitors, which may help to neutralize circulating virus and control the systemic inflammatory response associated with this disease.[51,55] However, FFP has been shown to be a poor means of supporting patient albumin concentrations, and very large volumes of plasma are required to achieve a small increase in plasma albumin.[55,64] Because of concern about transfusion-related immunomodulation and transfusion reactions, lack of efficacy, and readily available synthetic colloids, FFP is not recommended as a treatment to increase a patient's colloid oncotic pressure or serum albumin concentration.[64] There is a paucity of controlled clinical studies regarding albumin supplementation in veterinary patients, and to the authors' knowledge there have been no studies done to evaluate the efficacy of plasma transfusion for treatment in CPV enteritis. The administration of plasma as a means of providing passive immunization has been reported only anecdotally.[19,51] Despite these cautions and the paucity of studies evaluating the effect of FFP in CPV treatment, it is the experience of the authors that the early use of FFP has a positive effect on outcome.

Nil per os for 24 to 72 hours has been recommended in the past for the treatment of CPV enteritis. Growing evidence, however, supports the use of early enteral nutrition. A recent study has shown that puppies receiving early enteral nutrition via a nasoesophageal tube, when compared with puppies that received nil per os until vomiting ceased, showed earlier clinical improvement, significant weight gain, and improved gut barrier function, which could limit bacterial or endotoxin translocation.[66] Various commercial diets are formulated for animals recovering from gastrointestinal illness, but initial feeding should consist of small amounts of an easily digestible diet fed frequently even in the face of ongoing vomiting. The normal diet should be gradually introduced. Coinfection with intestinal parasites can exacerbate CPV enteritis by enhancing intestinal cell turnover and subsequent viral replication.[19] Appropriate oral therapy should be initiated as soon as vomiting ceases.

In dogs suffering from CPV enteritis, vomiting is most likely caused by destruction of intestinal crypt cells, abnormal intestinal motility, and endotoxin-induced activation of the cytokine cascade, leading to local irritation and central activation of the emetic center and chemoreceptor trigger zone.[67] Persistent vomiting leads to severe fluid and electrolyte loss, interferes with nutritional support, and precludes oral administration of medication. The most commonly used antiemetic drugs for CPV enteritis are metoclopramide, prochlorperazine, and ondansetron. Metoclopramide is a dopaminergic antagonist that blocks the chemoreceptor trigger zone, stimulates and coordinates motility of the upper intestinal tract, and increases pressure in the lower esophageal sphincter. Metoclopramide must be used with caution in patients at risk of intussusception. Prochlorperazine is a phenothiazine derivative that also limits stimulation of the chemoreceptor trigger zone. Ondansetron is a 5-HT3 receptor antagonist that acts peripherally and centrally to inhibit vomiting.[16,51,67] Of note, a retrospective study showed that in a high number of cases antiemetics did not completely control vomiting, and puppies that received antiemetics generally required longer hospitalization. It was concluded that, although sicker dogs (which have longer hospitalizations anyway) are more likely to require antiemetic drugs, complications of antiemetic drugs, such as hypotension, signs of depression, and immune modulation, could possibly contribute to extended periods of hospitalization. Although this study demonstrated an association between antiemetic use and prolonged hospitalization, a cause-and-effect conclusion cannot be drawn.[67] Antiemetics are definitely indicated in the management of this disease.

Treatment with intravenous, broad-spectrum, bactericidal antibiotics is warranted in puppies suffering from CPV enteritis due to the disruption of the intestinal barrier and severe leukopenia. A combination of a β-lactam antibiotic (ampicillin, 20 mg/kg intravenously [IV] every 8 hours) or a β-lactamase resistant penicillin (amoxicillin clavulanate, 20 mg/kg IV every 8 hours) with an aminoglycoside (amikacin, 20 mg/kg IV, intramuscularly, or subcutaneously every 24 hours once the dog has been rehydrated; used for a maximum of 5 days) will provide effective coverage.[16,51] The possibility does exist, however, that antibiotic therapy may increase the release of endotoxin and exacerbate the systemic inflammatory response.[31] Metronidazole (15–20 mg/kg by mouth every 12 hours for up to 10 days) is indicated in cases where protozoa are found on fecal wet prep.

Lately, more focus has been placed on immunotherapy for puppies suffering from CPV enteritis. The use of recombinant human G-CSF (rhG-CSF) has been investigated in puppies suffering from CPV enteritis with severe leukopenia.[44] To date investigators have not demonstrated benefit in puppies treated with rhG-CSF.[68,69] The ability of recombinant bactericidal/permeability-increasing protein ($rBPI_{21}$) to decrease plasma endotoxin concentration and severity of systemic clinical signs was investigated in CPV enteritis. Current data, however, do not show any benefit with its use.[70] Interferons (IFN) have the ability to modulate several cellular and immune functions, as well as affect virus replication.[71] Despite the lack of canine IFN products, several studies have shown recombinant feline interferon-ω (rFeIFN-ω) to significantly ameliorate severe enteritis caused by CPV and reduce mortality.[71–73] The benefit of oseltamivir, an antiviral drug that inhibits neuraminidase (NA), as a therapeutic agent in CPV was recently investigated. However, CPV does not rely on NA for replication, and the study showed no significant improvement in the days hospitalized or outcome of the patients.[74]

PREVENTION

Effective immunization protocols have been shown to be essential in the prevention of infection in susceptible puppies with CPV. Serum antibody titer is correlated with immunity. In mammals, antibodies are transferred to the neonate through the placenta and colostrum. These maternally derived antibodies play an important role in the protection of the neonate but are also considered one of the most important causes of immunization failures.[17,75] Based on hemagglutination-inhibition (HI) antibody titers, puppies receive approximately 90% of their total maternally derived CPV antibody from colostrum. Despite the low transplacental transfer of antibodies to CPV, the amount is still such that even colostrum-deprived puppies would be refractory to immunization or infection for several weeks. The amount of maternal antibody that puppies receive is proportional to the titer of the dam, and the amount of colostrum available to each puppy is inversely proportional to the size of the litter. Maternally derived antibody titers in puppies declines exponentially with time. The half-life of CPV maternal antibody was reported to be almost 10 days (9.7 days). The amount of maternally derived antibody that interferes with immunization is less than can be detected by the HI method, and the amount of antibody that will block active immunization is less than that necessary to prevent infection with street virus. Recovered animals maintain high antibody titers for at least 16 months after infection.[17]

Attenuated vaccines of canine origin, containing high-titer, low-passage CPV are currently the vaccines of choice. The term high titer refers to the amount of virus in the vaccine dose, and the term low passage refers to the number of times the virus was grown in various tissue cultures. Virus grown by fewer passages retains some of its ability to infect cells but does not cause disease.[2] Complete cross-protection has been reported between CPV-2, CPV-2a, and CPV-2b. The currently accepted vaccination protocol for CPV, based on data generated by vaccine manufacturers and individual researchers, recommends 3 doses of vaccine given at 6, 9, and 12 weeks of age.[75–77] Good protection has also been achieved with the use of a modified live CPV-2b vaccine administered intranasally.[78] Whether annual boosting is needed is controversial. Available data show that 93.7% of vaccinated dogs showed adequate response after more than 2 years following vaccination.[79] Data from dogs that recovered from active infection suggest that immunity following infection is long-lived, perhaps even life-long.[76] Increased risk of immune-mediated disease associated with overvaccination should compel practitioners to base their decision to administer booster annually on serologic results. Skepticism exists on the efficacy of current vaccines as preventive measures for CPV-2c.[80] A recent small study did, however, show cross-protection of 2 modified live vaccines, one containing CPV-2 and the other CPV-2b, against the CPV-2c strain.[81]

Despite the effectiveness of vaccination, good hygienic practices in kennels, including vigilant disinfection of all exposed surfaces and personnel, is extremely important in the prevention of the spread of the disease. Like all parvoviruses, CPV-2 is extremely stable and resistant to adverse environmental influences and can persist on inanimate objects such as clothing, food pans, and cage floors, for 5 months or longer.[6,15,16] Many detergents and disinfectants fail to inactivate canine parvoviruses. Sodium hypochlorite (common household bleach) is an effective viricidal disinfectant if exposure to this disinfectant lasts at least 1 hour.[15]

SUMMARY

Despite ongoing research in CPV enteritis, an agent-specific treatment remains elusive and basic therapeutic principles for gastroenteritis are still applicable. The identification of several prognosticators has, however, made management of the disease more rewarding. Parvoviral enteritis remains a significant pathogen in canines, especially because of the virus's ability to cause not only local gastrointestinal injury but also a significant systemic inflammatory response. Although effective vaccination has decreased incidence and mortality, the emergence of a new subspecies has led to concern about the efficacy of current vaccination protocols and subsequently about the susceptibility of populations considered to be immune.

REFERENCES

1. Pollock RV. The parvoviruses. II. Canine parvovirus. Compend Contin Educ Pract Vet 1984;6(7):653–64.
2. Smith-Carr S, Macintire DK, Swango LJ. Canine parvovirus. Part I. Pathogenesis and vaccination. Compend Contin Educ Pract Vet 1997;19(2):125–33.
3. Lamm CG, Rezabek GB. Parvovirus infection in domestic companion animals. Vet Clin North Am Small Anim Pract 2008;38(4):837–50.
4. Pollock RV. The parvoviruses. I. Feline panleukopenia virus and mink enteritis virus. Compend Contin Educ Pract Vet 1984;6(3):227–41.
5. Binn LN, Lazar EC, Eddy GA, et al. Recovery and characterization of a minute virus of canines. Infect Immun 1970;1(5):503–8.
6. Pollock RV, Coyne MJ. Canine parvovirus. Vet Clin North Am Small Anim Pract 1993;23(3):555–68.
7. Parrish CR, Have P, Foreyt WJ, et al. The global spread and replacement of canine parvovirus strains. J Gen Virol 1988;69(5):1111–6.
8. Buonavoglia C, Martella V, Pratelli A, et al. Evidence for evolution of canine parvovirus type 2 in Italy. J Gen Virol 2001;82(12):3021–5.
9. Nakamura M, Tohya Y, Miyazawa T, et al. A novel antigenic variant of canine parvovirus from a Vietnamese dog. Arch Virol 2004;149(11):2261–9.
10. Decaro N, Martella V, Desario C, et al. First detection of canine parvovirus type 2c in pups with haemorrhagic enteritis in Spain. J Vet Med B Infect Dis Vet Public Health 2006;53(10):468–72.
11. Hong C, Decaro N, Desario C, et al. Occurrence of canine parvovirus type 2c in the United States. J Vet Diagn Invest 2007;19(5):535–9.
12. Pérez R, Francia L, Romero V, et al. First detection of canine parvovirus type 2c in South America. Vet Microbiol 2007;124(1):147–52.
13. Vieira MJ, Silva E, Oliveira J, et al. Canine parvovirus 2c infection in central Portugal. J Vet Diagn Invest 2008;20(4):488–91.
14. Decaro N, Desario C, Addie DD, et al. Molecular epidemiology of canine parvovirus, Europe. Emerg Infect Dis 2007;13(8):1222–4.
15. Hoskins JD. Update on canine parvoviral enteritis. Vet Med 1997;92(8):694–709.
16. Prittie J. Canine parvoviral enteritis: a review of diagnosis, management, and prevention. J Vet Emerg Crit Care 2004;14(3):167–76.
17. Pollock RV, Carmichael LE. Maternally derived immunity to canine parvovirus infection: transfer, decline, and interference with vaccination. J Am Vet Med Assoc 1982;180(1):37–42.
18. O'Brien SE. Serologic response of pups to the low-passage, modified-live canine parvovirus-2 component in a combination vaccine. J Am Vet Med Assoc 1994;204(8):1207–9.
19. Brunner CJ, Swango LJ. Canine parvovirus infection: effects on the immune system and factors that predispose to severe disease. Compend Contin Educ Pract Vet 1985;7(12):979–88.

20. Houston DM, Ribble CS, Head LL. Risk factors associated with parvovirus enteritis in dogs: 283 cases (1982-1991). J Am Vet Med Assoc 1996;208(4): 542–6.
21. Glickman LT, Domanski LM, Patronek GJ, et al. Breed-related risk factors for canine parvovirus enteritis. J Am Vet Med Assoc 1985;187(6):589–94.
22. Shakespeare AS. The incidence of gastroenteritis diagnosis among sick dogs presented to the Onderstepoort Veterinary Academic Hospital correlated with meteorological data. J S Afr Vet Assoc 1999;70(2):95–7.
23. Johnson RH, Smith JR. Epidemiology and pathogenesis of canine parvovirus. Aust Vet Pract 1983;13(1):31.
24. Macartney L, McCandlish IAP, Thompson H, et al. Canine parvovirus enteritis. 2. Pathogenesis. Vet Rec 1984;115(18):453–60.
25. Appel M, Meunier P, Pollock R, et al. Canine viral enteritis, a report to practitioners. Canine Pract 1980;7(4):22–36.
26. Meunier PC, Cooper BJ, Appel MJ, et al. Pathogenesis of canine parvovirus enteritis: sequential virus distribution and passive immunization studies. Vet Pathol 1985;22(6):617–24.
27. Meunier PC, Cooper BJ, Appel MJ, et al. Pathogenesis of canine parvovirus enteritis: the importance of viremia. Vet Pathol 1985;22(1):60–71.
28. Jacobs RM, Weiser MG, Hall RL, et al. Clinicopathologic features of canine parvoviral enteritis. J Am Anim Hosp Assoc 1980;16(6):809–14.
29. O'Sullivan G, Durham PJ, Smith JR, et al. Experimentally induced severe canine parvoviral enteritis. Aust Vet J 1984;61(1):1–4.
30. Black JW, Holscher MA, Powell HS, et al. Parvoviral enteritis and panleukopenia in dogs. Vet Med Small Anim Clin 1979;74(1):47–50.
31. Otto CM, Drobatz KJ, Soter C. Endotoxemia and tumor necrosis factor activity in dogs with naturally occurring parvoviral enteritis. J Vet Intern Med 1997;11(2): 65–70.
32. Macartney L, McCandlish IA, Thompson H, et al. Canine parvovirus enteritis 1: clinical, haematological and pathological features of experimental infection. Vet Rec 1984;115(9):201–10.
33. Robinson WF, Huxtable CR, Pass DA, et al. Clinical and electrocardiographic findings in suspected viral myocarditis of pups. Aust Vet J 1979;55(8):351–5.
34. Robinson WF, Huxtable CR, Pass DA. Canine parvoviral myocarditis: a morphological description of the natural disease. Vet Pathol 1980;17(3):282–93.
35. Turk J, Miller M, Brown T, et al. Coliform septicemia and pulmonary disease associated with canine parvoviral enteritis: 88 cases (1987-1988). J Am Vet Med Assoc 1990;196(5):771–3.
36. Isogai E, Isogai H, Onuma M, et al. Escherichia coli associated endotoxemia in dogs with parvovirus infection. Jpn J Vet Sci 1989;51(3):597–606.
37. Wessels BC, Gaffin SL. Anti-endotoxin immunotherapy for canine parvovirus endotoxaemia. J Small Anim Pract 1986;27(10):609–15.
38. Weiss DJ, Rashid J. The sepsis-coagulant axis: a review. J Vet Intern Med 1998; 12(5):317–24.
39. Stander N, Wagner WM, Goddard A, et al. Normal canine pediatric gastrointestinal ultrasonography. Vet Radiol Ultrasound 2010;51(1):75–8.
40. Stander N, Wagner WM, Goddard A, et al. Ultrasonographic appearance of canine parvoviral enteritis in puppies. Vet Radiol Ultrasound 2010;51(1):69–74.
41. Goddard A, Leisewitz AL, Christopher MM, et al. Prognostic usefulness of blood leukocyte changes in canine parvoviral enteritis. J Vet Intern Med 2008;22(2): 309–16.

42. Potgieter LN, Jones JB, Patton CS, et al. Experimental parvovirus infection in dogs. Can J Comp Med 1981;45(3):212–6.
43. Boosinger TR, Rebar AH, DeNicola DB, et al. Bone marrow alterations associated with canine parvoviral enteritis. Vet Pathol 1982;19(5):558–61.
44. Cohn LA, Rewerts JM, McCaw D, et al. Plasma granulocyte colony-stimulating factor concentrations in neutropenic, parvoviral enteritis-infected puppies. J Vet Intern Med 1999;13(6):581–6.
45. Panda D, Patra RC, Nandi S, et al. Oxidative stress indices in gastroenteritis in dogs with canine parvoviral infection. Res Vet Sci 2009;86(1):36–42.
46. Wilson JJ, Neame PB, Kelton JG. Infection-induced thrombocytopenia. Semin Thromb Hemost 1982;8(3):217–33.
47. Axthelm MK, Krakowka S. Canine distemper virus-induced thrombocytopenia. Am J Vet Res 1987;48(8):1269–75.
48. Otto CM, Rieser TM, Brooks MB, et al. Evidence of hypercoagulability in dogs with parvoviral enteritis. J Am Vet Med Assoc 2000;217(10):1500–4.
49. Schoeman JP, Goddard A, Herrtage ME. Serum cortisol and thyroxine concentrations as predictors of death in critically ill puppies with parvoviral diarrhea. J Am Vet Med Assoc 2007;231(10):1534–9.
50. Schoeman JP, Herrtage ME. Serum thyrotropin, thyroxine and free thyroxine concentrations as predictors of mortality in critically ill puppies with parvovirus infection: a model for human paediatric critical illness? Microbes Infect 2008; 10(2):203–7.
51. Macintire DK, Smith-Carr S. Canine parvovirus. Part II. Clinical signs, diagnosis, and treatment. Compend Contin Educ Pract Vet 1997;19(3):291–302.
52. Heald RD, Jones BD, Schmidt DA. Blood gas and electrolyte concentrations in canine parvoviral enteritis. J Am Anim Hosp Assoc 1986;22(6):745–8.
53. Mann FA, Boon GD, Wagner-Mann C, et al. Ionized and total magnesium concentrations in blood from dogs with naturally acquired parvoviral enteritis. J Am Vet Med Assoc 1998;212(9):1398–401.
54. Broek AH. Serum protein electrophoresis in canine parvovirus enteritis. Br Vet J 1990;146(3):255–9.
55. Mazzaferro EM, Rudloff E, Kirby R. The role of albumin replacement in the critically ill veterinary patient. J Vet Emerg Crit Care 2002;12(2):113–24.
56. Yilmaz Z, Senturk S. Characterisation of lipid profiles in dogs with parvoviral enteritis. J Small Anim Pract 2007;48(11):643–50.
57. Rai A, Nauriyal DC. A note on acid-base status and blood gas dynamics in canine parvo viral gastroenteritis. Indian J Vet Med 1992;12(2):87–8.
58. Nappert G, Dunphy E, Ruben D, et al. Determination of serum organic acids in puppies with naturally acquired parvoviral enteritis. Can J Vet Res 2002;66(1): 15–8.
59. Pollock RV, Carmichael LE. Canine viral enteritis. In: Barlough JE, editor. Manual of small animal infectious diseases. New York: Churchill Livingston; 1988. p. 101–7.
60. Helfer-Baker C, Evermann JF, McKeirnan AJ, et al. Serological studies on the incidence of canine enteritis viruses. Canine Pract 1980;7(3):37–42.
61. Mohan R, Nauriyal DC, Singh KB. Detection of canine parvo virus in faeces, using a parvo virus ELISA test kit. Indian Vet J 1993;70(4):301–3.
62. Desario C, Decaro N, Campolo M, et al. Canine parvovirus infection: which diagnostic test for virus? J Virol Methods 2005;126(1):179–85.
63. JinSik O, GunWoo H, YoungShik C, et al. One-step immunochromatography assay kit for detecting antibodies to canine parvovirus. Clin Vaccine Immunol 2006;13(4):520–4.

64. Brown AJ, Otto CM. Fluid therapy in vomiting and diarrhea. Vet Clin North Am Small Anim Pract 2008;38(3):653–75.
65. Lobetti RG, Joubert KE, Picard J, et al. Bacterial colonization of intravenous catheters in young dogs suspected to have parvoviral enteritis. J Am Vet Med Assoc 2002;220(9):1321–4.
66. Mohr AJ, Leisewitz AL, Jacobson LS, et al. Effect of early enteral nutrition on intestinal permeability, intestinal protein loss, and outcome in dogs with severe parvoviral enteritis. J Vet Intern Med 2003;17(6):791–8.
67. Mantione NL, Otto CM. Characterization of the use of antiemetic agents in dogs with parvoviral enteritis treated at a veterinary teaching hospital: 77 cases (1997-2000). J Am Vet Med Assoc 2005;227(11):1787–93.
68. Rewerts JM, McCaw DL, Cohn LA, et al. Recombinant human granulocyte colony-stimulating factor for treatment of puppies with neutropenia secondary to canine parvovirus infection. J Am Vet Med Assoc 1998;213(7):991–2.
69. Mischke R, Barth T, Wohlsein P, et al. Effect of recombinant human granulocyte colony-stimulating factor (rhG-CSF) on leukocyte count and survival rate of dogs with parvoviral enteritis. Res Vet Sci 2001;70(3):221–5.
70. Otto CM, Jackson CB, Rogell EJ, et al. Recombinant bactericidal/permeability-increasing protein (rBPI$_{21}$) for treatment of parvovirus enteritis: a randomized, double-blinded, placebo-controlled trial. J Vet Intern Med 2001;15(4):355–60.
71. Ishiwata K, Minagawa T, Kajimoto T. Clinical effects of the recombinant feline interferon-ω on experimental parvovirus infection in Beagle dogs. J Vet Med Sci 1998;60(8):911–7.
72. Martin V, Najbar W, Gueguen S, et al. Treatment of canine parvoviral enteritis with interferon-omega in a placebo-controlled challenge trial. Vet Microbiol 2002; 89(2):115–27.
73. Mari K, Maynard L, Eun HM, et al. Treatment of canine parvoviral enteritis with interferon-omega in a placebo-controlled field trial. Vet Rec 2003;152(4):105–8.
74. Savigny MR, Macintire DK. Use of oseltamivir in the treatment of canine parvoviral enteritis. J Vet Emerg Crit Care 2010;20(1):132–42.
75. Waner T, Naveh A, Wudovsky I, et al. Assessment of maternal antibody decay and response to canine parvovirus vaccination using a clinic-based enzyme-linked immunosorbent assay. J Vet Diagn Invest 1996;8(4):427–32.
76. Buonavoglia C, Tollis M, Buonavoglia D, et al. Response of pups with maternal derived antibody to modified-live canine parvovirus vaccine. Comp Immunol Microbiol Infect Dis 1992;15(4):281–3.
77. Bergman JG, Muniz M, Sutton D, et al. Comparative trial of the canine parvovirus, canine distemper virus and canine adenovirus type 2 fractions of two commercially available modified live vaccines. Vet Rec 2006;159(22):733–6.
78. Martella V, Cavalli A, Decaro N, et al. Immunogenicity of an intranasally administered modified live canine parvovirus type 2b vaccine in pups with maternally derived antibodies. Clin Diagn Lab Immunol 2005;12(10):1243–5.
79. Twark L, Dodds WJ. Clinical use of serum parvovirus and distemper virus antibody titers for determining revaccination strategies in healthy dogs. J Am Vet Med Assoc 2000;217(7):1021–4.
80. Kapil S, Cooper E, Lamm C, et al. Canine parvovirus types 2c and 2b circulating in North American dogs in 2006 and 2007. J Clin Microbiol 2007;45(12):4044–7.
81. Larson LJ, Schultz RD. Do two current canine parvovirus type 2 and 2b vaccines provide protection against the new type 2c variant? Vet Ther 2008;9(2):94–101.

Antiviral Therapy for Feline Herpesvirus Infections

David J. Maggs, BVSc (Hons)

KEYWORDS

• Herpesvirus • Feline • Virology • Antiviral therapy
• Pharmacology

A large variety of antiviral agents exists for oral or topical (ophthalmic) treatment of cats infected with feline herpesvirus type 1 (FHV-1). However, some general comments regarding these agents are possible. Knowledge of these general principles can be used to better understand antiviral pharmacology and thereby guide therapy for cats with herpetic disease.

- No antiviral agent has been developed specifically for FHV-1, although many have been tested for efficacy against this virus. Agents highly effective against closely related human herpesviruses (for which they were developed) are not necessarily or predictably effective against FHV-1 and all should be tested in vitro before they are administered to cats. In vitro potency is described as the drug concentration at which viral replication is suppressed by 50% (or IC_{50}). Therefore, a more potent drug will have a lower IC_{50}. **Table 1** summarizes the relative antiviral efficacy against FHV-1 and human herpes simplex virus type 1 (HSV-1) for a number of antiviral drugs.
- No antiviral agent has been developed specifically for cats; although some have been tested for safety in this species. Agents with a reasonable safety profile in humans are not always or predictably nontoxic when administered to cats and all require safety and efficacy testing in vivo.
- Many systemically and topically administered antiviral agents require host and or viral metabolism before achieving their active form. These agents are not reliably or predictably metabolized by cats or FHV-1 and pharmacokinetic studies in cats and in vitro efficacy testing are required.

Work reported here was supported in part by the UC Davis Center for Comparative Animal Health, The American College of Veterinary Ophthalmologists, Vision for Animals Foundation, The Morris Animal Foundation, Winn Feline Foundation, The George and Phyllis Miller Feline Health Fund, Ralston Purina Company, and the Toots Fund.
Department of Surgical and Radiological Sciences, School of Veterinary Medicine, University of California-Davis, One Shields Avenue, Davis, CA 95616, USA
E-mail address: djmaggs@ucdavis.edu

Table 1
Comparative antiviral efficacy (expressed as IC_{50}) against FHV-1 and HSV-1 for various antiviral compounds

IC_{50} (μM)	TFU	GCV	IDU	CDV	PCV	VDB	ACV	Foscarnet
FHV-1	$1\text{-}19^{1,2}$	5^3	$4\text{-}7^{1,3}$	$8\text{-}168^{3-5}$	$1\text{-}130^{3-5}$	21^1	$16\text{-}222^{1-6}$	233^3
HSV-1	1.7	0.8	1	9	2	4	1	74

Abbreviations: ACV, acyclovir; CDV, cidofovir; GCV, ganciclovir; IDU, idoxuridine; μM, micromolar; PCV, penciclovir; TFU, trifluridine; VDB, vidarabine.

- Antiviral agents tend to be more toxic than do antibacterial agents because viruses are obligate intracellular organisms and co-opt or have close analogs of the host's cellular "machinery." This limits many antiviral agents to topical (ophthalmic) rather than systemic use. For those which can be administered systemically, a relatively narrow safety margin often exists and special considerations should always be given to patients with reduced hepatic or renal function.
- All antiviral agents currently used for cats infected with FHV-1 are virostatic. Therefore, they typically require frequent administration to be effective and must be understood to merely retard viral growth while the host immune response clears the virus.

The following antiviral agents have been studied to varying degrees for their efficacy against FHV-1, their pharmacokinetics in cats, or their safety and efficacy in treating cats infected with FHV-1.

IDOXURIDINE

Idoxuridine is a thymidine analog originally developed for treatment of humans infected with HSV-1. Following intracellular phosphorylation, it competes with thymidine for incorporation into viral DNA, rendering the resultant virus incapable of replication. However, it apparently does this less effectively in FHV-1 than in HSV-1 (see **Table 1**). In addition, idoxuridine is a nonspecific inhibitor of DNA synthesis, affecting any process requiring thymidine. Therefore, host cells are similarly affected, systemic therapy is not possible, and corneal toxicity can occur. It has historically been commercially available as an ophthalmic 0.1% solution or 0.5% ointment, but is no longer commercially available in the United States. It can be obtained from a compounding pharmacist in these forms and is well tolerated by most cats and seems efficacious in many. It should be applied to the affected eye five to six times daily.

VIDARABINE

Vidarabine is an adenosine analog that, following triphosphorylation, appears to affect viral DNA synthesis by interfering with DNA polymerase. However, like idoxuridine, vidarabine is nonselective in its effect and so is associated with notable host toxicity if administered systemically. Because it affects a viral replication step different from that targeted by idoxuridine, vidarabine may be effective in patients whose disease seems resistant to idoxuridine. Where it is not available commercially, it can be obtained from a compounding pharmacist as a 3% ophthalmic ointment. Anecdotal reports suggest that vidarabine may be better tolerated by cats than many of the antiviral solutions. Like idoxuridine, it should be applied to the affected eye five to six times daily.

TRIFLURIDINE

Like idoxuridine, trifluridine is a nucleoside analog of thymidine. However, it is believed to have a somewhat different mode of action. Following intracellular phosphorylation it is presumed to reduce DNA synthesis via inhibition of thymidylate synthase. It is too toxic to be administered systemically but topically administered trifluridine is considered one of the most effective drugs for treating HSV-1 keratitis. This is in part due to its superior corneal epithelial penetration.[7] It is also one of the more potent antiviral drugs for FHV-1 (see **Table 1**). It is commercially available in the United States as a 1% ophthalmic solution that should be applied to the affected eye five to six times daily. Unfortunately, it is expensive and is often not well tolerated by cats, presumably due to a stinging reaction reported in humans.

ACYCLOVIR

Acyclovir is the prototype of a group of antiviral drugs known as acyclic nucleoside analogs. Members of this group of antiviral agents all require three phosphorylation steps for activation. The first of these steps must be catalyzed by a viral enzyme, thymidine kinase. This fact increases their safety and permits them to be systemically administered to humans. However, the activity of this enzyme in FHV-1 is not equivalent to that in HSV-1.[8] The second and third phosphorylation steps must be performed by host enzymes, which may not be present in cats or may not be as effective in cats as they are in humans. This knowledge helps explain why the acyclic nucleoside antiviral agents developed for humans infected with HSV-1 are not predictably safe or effective when administered to cats infected with FHV-1 and why pharmacokinetic studies are always needed to establish appropriate dosing in cats. In addition to relatively low antiviral potency against FHV-1, acyclovir has poor bioavailability in cats and is potentially toxic when systemically administered.[9] Oral administration of 50 mg/kg acyclovir to cats was associated with peak plasma levels of approximately only one-third the IC_{50} for this virus (33 μM).[9] Common signs of toxicity are referable to bone marrow suppression. In some countries, acyclovir is also available as a 3% ophthalmic ointment. In one study in which a 0.5% ointment was used five times daily, the median time to resolution of clinical signs was 10 days.[2] Cats treated only three times daily took approximately twice as long to resolve and did so only once therapy was increased to five times daily. Taken together, these data suggest that very frequent topical application of acyclovir may produce concentrations at the corneal surface that do exceed the reported IC_{50} for this virus but are not associated with toxicity. There are also in vitro data suggesting that interferon exerts a synergistic effect with acyclovir that could permit an approximately eightfold reduction in acyclovir dose.[10] In vivo investigation and validation of these data are needed.

VALACYCLOVIR

Valacyclovir is an acyclic nucleoside analog and a prodrug of acyclovir that, in humans and cats, is more efficiently absorbed from the gastrointestinal tract compared with acyclovir and is converted to acyclovir by a hepatic hydrolase. Its safety and efficacy have been studied in cats.[11] Plasma concentrations of acyclovir that surpass the IC_{50} for FHV-1 can be achieved after oral administration of valacyclovir. However, in cats experimentally infected with FHV-1, valacyclovir induced fatal hepatic and renal necrosis, along with bone marrow suppression, and did not reduce viral shedding or clinical disease severity.[11] Therefore, despite its superior pharmacokinetics, valacyclovir should never be used in cats.

GANCICLOVIR

Ganciclovir is another acyclic nucleoside analog that also requires triphosphorylation to achieve its active form. Like acyclovir, the first phosphorylation step is mediated by viral thymidine kinase. Despite these similarities, it appears to be at least 10-fold more effective than is acyclovir against FHV-1 suggesting a relative difference in cellular drug uptake, rate, or efficacy of host or viral phosphorylation,[4,8] metabolite stability, or mode of action of these two drugs.[3] Ganciclovir is available for systemic (intravenous or by mouth) and intravitreal administration in humans, where it is associated with greater toxicity than acyclovir. Toxicity is typically evident as bone marrow suppression. Very recently, a 0.15% ophthalmic gel formulation of ganciclovir has become available for humans infected with HSV-1. Ganciclovir holds promise for feline herpetic disease and currently available formulations warrant safety and efficacy studies in cats.

PENCICLOVIR

Penciclovir is a nucleoside deoxyguanosine analog with a similar mechanism of action as acyclovir and potent antiviral activity for a number of human herpesviruses. It too requires viral and cellular phosphorylation and yet has relatively high antiviral efficacy against FHV-1, due at least in part to the efficiency with which this drug is phosphorylated by FHV-1 thymidine kinase.[8] It is available as a dermatologic cream for humans that should not be applied to the eye. We have some preliminary data in which we administered PCV intravenously to cats, but this was done largely to assist with our ongoing investigations of the penciclovir prodrug, famciclovir (Thomasy SM and colleagues, unpublished data, 2008). In vivo studies of the safety or efficacy of penciclovir in cats are otherwise lacking and, at this time, its use in cats cannot be recommended.

FAMCICLOVIR

Famciclovir is a prodrug of penciclovir; however, metabolism of famciclovir to penciclovir is complex and requires di-deacetylation, predominantly in the blood, and subsequent oxidation to penciclovir by a hepatic aldehyde oxidase. Unfortunately, the activity of this hepatic aldehyde oxidase is negligible in cats.[12] This necessitates cautious extrapolation to cats of data generated in humans. Data to date in normal and experimentally infected cats suggest that the pharmacokinetics of this drug are extremely complex and likely result from nonlinear famciclovir absorption, metabolism, excretion, or an combination of these three factors.[13,14] In spite this, there is mounting evidence that suggests famciclovir is very effective in some cats with experimentally induced or suspected spontaneous herpetic disease.[15–19] Further studies of this drug's pharmacokinetics, safety, and efficacy are required before dose rates and frequency can be recommended.

CIDOFOVIR

Cidofovir is a relatively new cytosine analog that requires the typical two host-mediated phosphorylation steps without virally mediated phosphorylation. Its safety arises from its relatively high affinity for HSV DNA polymerase compared with human DNA polymerase.[20] It is commercially available only in injectable form in the United States, but has been studied as a 0.5% solution applied topically twice daily to cats experimentally infected with FHV-1.[21] Its use in these cats was associated with reduced viral shedding and clinical disease.[21] Its efficacy at only twice daily (despite being virostatic) is believed to be due to the long tissue half-lives of the metabolites of this drug.[22] There are reports of its experimental topical use in humans and rabbits being associated with stenosis of the nasolacrimal drainage system components and, as yet, it is not commercially available as an ophthalmic agent in humans.[23,24] Therefore, although extremely effective in cats, at this stage there are insufficient data to support its long term safety as a topical agent.

LYSINE

There is an expanding amount of literature regarding use of lysine as a therapy for cats with herpetic disease. Although the safety of this approach has not been questioned, there are some variable efficacy data.

IN VITRO EFFICACY AGAINST FHV-1

Lysine limits the in vitro replication of many viruses, including FHV-1. The antiviral mechanism is unknown; however, many investigators have demonstrated that concurrent depletion of arginine is essential for lysine supplementation to be effective. This finding suggests that lysine exerts its antiviral effect by antagonism of arginine. This is also true for FHV-1 where arginine is an essential amino acid for viral replication but, in the presence of small amounts of arginine, lysine supplementation reduces viral replication by about 50%.[25] However, this effect was not seen in media containing higher arginine concentrations, suggesting that a high lysine/arginine ratio is critical for efficacy.

IN VIVO EFFICACY IN CATS

Results of two early independent in vivo studies supported the clinical use of lysine in cats. In the first of these studies,[26] eight FHV-1–naive cats were administered 500 mg of lysine orally every 12 hours beginning 6 hours before, and continuing for 3 weeks after, experimental inoculation with FHV-1. Lysine-treated cats had significantly less severe conjunctivitis than cats that received placebo. In the second study,[27] 14 cats latently infected with FHV-1 received 400 mg of lysine per os every 24 hours. Viral shedding was monitored for 30 days. Lysine administration in these cats was associated with a statistically significant reduction in basal viral shedding compared with cats that received placebo. Since these cats were normal, latently infected carrier cats, little or no clinical disease was seen during the month-long study in the placebo or lysine group. In both studies, plasma arginine concentrations remained in the normal range, and no signs of toxicity were observed, despite notably elevated plasma lysine concentrations in treated cats. Both of these studies used experimentally infected line-bred cats. Therefore, the applicability of these data in naturally infected, genetically diverse cats required investigation.

A subsequent study examined the effects of lysine in 144 cats residing in a humane shelter.[28] Cats received oral boluses of 250 mg (kittens) or 500 mg (adult cats) of lysine once daily for the duration of their stay at the shelter and outcomes were compared with those of an untreated control group. No significant treatment effect was detected on the incidence of infectious upper respiratory disease (IURD), the need for antimicrobial treatment for IURD, or the interval from admission to onset of IURD. However it was not determined if and to what extent these cats were shedding or infected with FHV-1 or other pathogens. This study also highlights the concern that daily handling of cats for bolus administration of lysine may not only be ineffective but actually stimulate further viral reactivation through stress or cause transfer of pathogens between cats by shelter workers administering the lysine. Therefore studies examining the safety and efficacy of lysine incorporated into cat food were conducted. An initial safety trial[29] revealed that cats fed a diet supplemented with up to 8.6% achieved plasma lysine concentrations similar to those achieved with bolus administration, showed no signs of toxicity, and had normal plasma arginine concentrations. In a subsequent study,[30] 50 cats with enzootic IURD were fed a basal diet ($\sim$1% lysine) or a diet supplemented to approximately 5% lysine for 52 days while subjected to rehousing stress, which is known to cause viral reactivation.[31] Perhaps not unexpectedly, food (and, therefore, lysine) intake decreased coincident with peak disease and viral presence. As a result, cats did not receive additional lysine at the very time they needed it most. Analysis of the data revealed that disease in cats fed the supplemented ration was more severe than that in cats fed the basal diet. In addition, viral shedding was more frequent in cats receiving the supplemented diet.[30]

To further elucidate the efficacy of dietary lysine supplementation, we performed a similarly designed experiment[32] in a local humane shelter with a more consistent "background" level of stress and with greater numbers enrolled compared with the initial rehousing study.[30] We enrolled 261 cats; each for 4 weeks. Despite plasma lysine concentration in treated cats being greater than that in control cats, more treated cats than control cats developed moderate to severe disease and shed FHV-1 DNA at certain points throughout the study.

Unfortunately, there is considerable variability among all of these studies of lysine safety and efficacy, especially with respect to methodology, study population, and dose and method of lysine administration. Taken together, data from these studies seem to suggest that lysine is safe when orally administered to cats and, when administered as a bolus, may reduce viral shedding in latently infected cats and clinical signs in cats undergoing primary exposure to the virus. However, the stress of bolus administration in shelter situations may well negate its effects and data do not support dietary supplementation. Unfortunately, no studies to date have been conducted on client-owned cats although anecdotal evidence suggests that there is a benefit from administration of lysine. Although each clinical presentation needs to be assessed individually, I recommend that lysine be administered to client-owned cats as a twice daily (500 mg) bolus and not added to food. Owners should be made aware that this is usually only an adjunctive or palliative therapy and that administration of antiviral drugs may also be necessary to gain better control of signs. Unlike the protocol for HSV-1-infected humans, owners of cats receiving lysine for FHV-1 should not be advised to restrict their cat's arginine intake.

SUMMARY

Data generated in recent in vitro and in vivo studies have provided much support for the use of antiviral drugs as well as the amino acid lysine. Although these populations provide numerous advantages for initial studies of drug safety and efficacy, it is important to interpret these data in light of the populations in which they were generated. It is likely that data gained from treating laboratory-bred, experimentally-infected animals need not always apply directly to more genetically diverse naturally infected cats. It is to be hoped that well designed, placebo-controlled, double-masked studies in client owned animals will be forthcoming.

REFERENCES

1. Nasisse MP, Guy JS, Davidson MG, et al. In vitro susceptibility of feline herpesvirus-1 to vidarabine, idoxuridine, trifluridine, acyclovir, or bromovinyldeoxyuridine. Am J Vet Res 1989;50(1):158–60.

2. Williams DL, Robinson JC, Lay E, et al. Efficacy of topical aciclovir for the treatment of feline herpetic keratitis: results of a prospective clinical trial and data from in vitro investigations. Vet Rec 2005;157(9):254–7.
3. Maggs DJ, Clarke HE. In vitro efficacy of ganciclovir, cidofovir, penciclovir, foscarnet, idoxuridine, and acyclovir against feline herpesvirus type-1. Am J Vet Res 2004;65(4):399–403.
4. Hussein IT, Menashy RV, Field HJ. Penciclovir is a potent inhibitor of feline herpesvirus-1 with susceptibility determined at the level of virus-encoded thymidine kinase. Antiviral Res 2008;78(3):268–74.
5. Hussein IT, Field HJ. Development of a quantitative real-time TaqMan PCR assay for testing the susceptibility of feline herpesvirus-1 to antiviral compounds. J Virol Methods 2008;152(1–2):85–90.
6. Collins P. The spectrum of antiviral activities of acyclovir in vitro and in vivo. J Antimicrob Chemother 1983;12(Suppl B):19–27.
7. Pavan-Langston D, Nelson DJ. Intraocular penetration of trifluridine. Am J Ophthalmol 1979;87(6):814–8.
8. Hussein IT, Miguel RN, Tiley LS, et al. Substrate specificity and molecular modelling of the feline herpesvirus-1 thymidine kinase. Arch Virol 2008;153(3):495–505.
9. Owens JG, Nasisse MP, Tadepalli SM, et al. Pharmacokinetics of acyclovir in the cat. J Vet Pharmacol Ther 1996;19(6):488–90.
10. Weiss RC. Synergistic antiviral activities of acyclovir and recombinant human leukocyte (alpha) interferon on feline herpesvirus replication. Am J Vet Res 1989;50(10):1672–7.
11. Nasisse MP, Dorman DC, Jamison KC, et al. Effects of valacyclovir in cats infected with feline herpesvirus 1. Am J Vet Res 1997;58(10):1141–4.
12. Dick RA, Kanne DB, Casida JE. Identification of aldehyde oxidase as the neonicotinoid nitroreductase. Chem Res Toxicol 2005;18(2):317–23.
13. Thomasy SM, Maggs DJ, Moulin NK, et al. Pharmacokinetics and safety of penciclovir following oral administration of famciclovir to cats. Am J Vet Res 2007; 68(11):1252–8.
14. Thomasy SM, Whittem T, Stanley SD, et al. Pharmacokinetics of famciclovir and penciclovir following single-dose oral administration of famciclovir to cats. Vet Ophthalmol 2009;12(6):402.
15. Thomasy SM, Maggs DJ, Lim CC, et al. Safety and efficacy of famciclovir in cats infected with feline herpesvirus 1. Vet Ophthalmol 2007;10(6):418.
16. Malik R, Lessels NS, Webb S, et al. Treatment of feline herpesvirus-1 associated disease in cats with famciclovir and related drugs. J Feline Med Surg 2009;11(1): 40–8.
17. Thomasy SM, Maggs DJ. Treatment of ocular nasal, and dermatologic disease attributable to feline herpesvirus 1 with famciclovir. Vet Ophthalmol 2008;11(6): 418.
18. Thomasy SM, Lim CC, Reilly CM, et al. Safety and efficacy of orally administered famciclovir in cats experimentally infected with feline herpesvirus 1. Am J Vet Res, in press.
19. Lim CC, Reilly CM, Thomasy SM, et al. Effects of famciclovir on tear film parameters in cats experimentally infected with feline herpesvirus 1. Am J Vet Res 2009; 70(3):394–403.
20. Neyts J, Snoeck R, Schols D, et al. Selective inhibition of human cytomegalovirus DNA synthesis by (S)-1-(3-hydroxy-2-phosphonylmethoxypropyl)cytosine [(S)-HPMPC] and 9-(1,3-dihydroxy-2-propoxymethyl)guanine (DHPG). Virology 1990;179(1):41–50.

21. Fontenelle JP, Powell CC, Veir JK, et al. Effect of topical ophthalmic application of cidofovir on experimentally induced primary ocular feline herpesvirus-1 infection in cats. Am J Vet Res 2008;69(2):289–93.

22. Neyts J, Snoeck R, Balzarini J, et al. Particular characteristics of the anti-human cytomegalovirus activity of (S)-1-(3-hydroxy-2-phosphonylmethoxypropyl)cytosine (HPMPC) in vitro. Antiviral Res 1991;16(1):41–52.

23. Sherman MD, Feldman KA, Farahmand SM, et al. Treatment of conjunctival squamous cell carcinoma with topical cidofovir. Am J Ophthalmol 2002;134(3):432–3.

24. Inoue H, Sonoda KH, Ishikawa M, et al. Clinical evaluation of local ocular toxicity in candidate anti-adenoviral agents in vivo. Ophthalmologica 2009;223(4):233–8.

25. Maggs DJ, Collins BK, Thorne JG, et al. Effects of L-lysine and L-arginine on in vitro replication of feline herpesvirus type-1. Am J Vet Res 2000;61(12):1474–8.

26. Stiles J, Townsend WM, Rogers QR, et al. Effect of oral administration of L-lysine on conjunctivitis caused by feline herpesvirus in cats. Am J Vet Res 2002;63(1):99–103.

27. Maggs DJ, Nasisse MP, Kass PH. Efficacy of oral supplementation with L-lysine in cats latently infected with feline herpesvirus. Am J Vet Res 2003;64(1):37–42.

28. Rees TM, Lubinski JL. Oral supplementation with L-lysine did not prevent upper respiratory infection in a shelter population of cats. J Feline Med Surg 2008;10(5):510–3.

29. Fascetti AJ, Maggs DJ, Kanchuk ML, et al. Excess dietary lysine does not cause lysine-arginine antagonism in adult cats. J Nutr 2004;134(Suppl 8):2042S–5S.

30. Maggs DJ, Sykes JE, Clarke HE, et al. Effects of dietary lysine supplementation in cats with enzootic upper respiratory disease. J Feline Med Surg 2007;9(2):97–108.

31. Gaskell RM, Povey RC. Experimental induction of feline viral rhinotracheitis virus re-excretion in FVR-recovered cats. Vet Rec 1977;100(7):128–33.

32. Drazenovich TL, Fascetti AJ, Westermeyer HD, et al. Effects of dietary lysine supplementation on upper respiratory and ocular disease and detection of infectious organisms in cats within an animal shelter. Am J Vet Res 2009;70(11):1391–400.

Canine Influenza

Edward J. Dubovi, PhD

KEYWORDS

• Canine • Influenza • Epidemiology • Diagnosis
• Treatment • Prevention

Canine influenza as a recognized clinical entity in dogs has a relatively brief history. There were a few early reports on the presence of antibodies to human influenza virus in dogs and the ability to induce an antibody response in dogs when challenged with the human influenza virus.[1,2] However, no clinical disease was linked to any natural or experimental exposures. This scenario changed mainly as a result of 2 events. The emergence of the highly pathogenic avian influenza virus H5N1 in Southeast Asia in 1996-1997 focused public health efforts on the potential of a new pandemic of human influenza. Funding became available for enhanced surveillance programs and validation of molecular testing that could detect virtually any strain of influenza virus regardless of the hemagglutinin (HA) subtype. Although the focus in the animal world was mainly on migrating wild birds as vehicles for the spread of the virus to distant regions, any animal with respiratory signs became a target for testing. The relative ease of testing with reverse transcriptase-polymerase chain reaction (RT-PCR) technology has expanded surveillance at all levels.

The second event that defined the beginning of canine influenza was the isolation of an influenza virus from racing greyhounds that experienced moderate to severe respiratory infections in early 2004.[3] This report focused the canine world on the possibility that the influenza virus was a contributor to the acute respiratory disease complex in canines. Subsequent data showed that this virus had a unique genetic signature that defined a new entity known as canine influenza virus (CIV).[3,4]

With the introduction of the term CIV, there is a need to define the nomenclature that is used in this review. Canine influenza is used to note the disease in dogs induced by any influenza virus infection. CIV is reserved for those viruses that have a defined genetic signature that sets them apart from their progenitor virus. All influenza viruses originated in avian species, but with time some have become established in an alternative host. Most pertinent for this discussion is the entity H3N8 equine influenza virus (EIV). Although this virus is most certainly of avian origin, association with the equine host has brought about sequence changes that clearly define a virus that is separate

The author has nothing to disclose.
Department of Population and Diagnostic Sciences, Animal Health Diagnostic Center, College of Veterinary Medicine, Cornell University, Ithaca, NY 14853, USA
E-mail address: ejd5@cornell.edu

from the H3N8 virus circulating in birds at present. The first influenza virus isolated from clinically ill dogs was an H3N8 of equine origin. However, the virus does have a genetic signature related to the HA protein that distinguishes it from the equine progenitor.[3,4] CIV is defined as unique not only by genetic changes but also by the biologic difference of not being able to establish a productive infection in experimentally challenged horses (Landolt GA, Colorado Springs, CO, personal communication, May 2010.) CIV in this article is used exclusively for the genetically distinct H3N8 virus isolated in canines in the United States. As more genetic information becomes available on viruses isolated from canines, this nomenclature may need to be changed to account for the multiple H and N (ie, hemagglutinin and neuraminidase) subtypes linked to canine influenza.

Even though canine influenza is a new clinical entity in dogs, 4 review articles on canine influenza have been published in the last few years.[5–8]

H3N8

The official beginning of canine influenza was with the identification of an influenza virus in cases of respiratory disease in greyhounds in the racing industry of the United States in March 2004.[3] For several years preceding this discovery, the racing industry had been plagued by frequent outbreaks of respiratory disease that caused significant economic losses despite standard prevention methods including vaccination. Attempts to identify the cause of these outbreaks failed to consistently identify an agent that could be linked to the acute respiratory disease cases. With the identification of influenza virus associated with one outbreak, serologic testing on other animals linked to the racing industry quickly determined that the exposure to what became known as the CIV was widespread. Additional isolates from greyhounds were identified in Texas in July 2004[3] and Iowa in April 2005.[9]

Although the finding of CIV in racing greyhounds was a significant event, an important question was whether this virus would find its way into the companion animal population. In 2005, both virus isolations and serologic data confirmed that CIV had moved into companion animals in Florida and the New York City area.[4,5] This discovery was followed in early 2006 with the identification of the virus in the Denver, Colorado area. Transmission of CIV from dog to dog was clearly involved in these cases, indicating a new cross-species jump of influenza virus.

Sequence analysis of the initial CIV isolate indicated that it was most closely related to EIV H3N8.[3,4] All 8 gene segments were of equine origin, so no gene reassortment was responsible for the infection in dogs. Even with the earliest CIV isolates, there were amino acid changes in the HA protein that distinguished CIV from the EIVs circulating in the United States. Questions concerning the origin of this virus and its genetic drift became active areas of interest. To date, all CIV isolates examined belong to a single lineage, that is, the data point to a single introduction of a unique variant of EIV (Donis RO, Atlanta, GA, personal communication, June 2010.)[3,4] These analyses include CIV isolates from Florida, New York, Colorado, and all areas into which CIV was carried from these 3 enzootic areas. As with all influenza viruses, genetic drift is occurring as the virus continues to circulate in dogs. There is some suggestion that should the virus continue to circulate, unique clades may develop that are linked to the geographic centers of infection, not unlike what has happened with EIV.

The exact geographic origin of CIV will never be known, and its initial isolation in Florida may have been unrelated to the site of the initial transmission from a horse to a dog. Best estimates are that this event may have occurred in 1999–2000. No

CIV isolates exist before 2003, and serologic data may not be of help because of the ability of EIV to infect dogs. The key biologic difference between EIV and CIV is the ability of CIV to be transmitted from dog to dog. Experimental infections have clearly shown transmissibility of CIV.[10] Some confusion was caused by reports of the presence of antibodies to CIV in dogs in the United Kingdom.[11] It soon became evident that EIV could infect dogs, but the virus was not transmitted beyond the initial focus of infection. This discovery was confirmed during the large epizootic outbreak of EIV in Australia in 2007, where EIV was transmitted to dogs from horses on the affected farms. The infections were detected by RT-PCR and serology, but no evidence of transmission to contact dogs was found.[12] Experimentally, EIV was transmitted from infected horses to in-contact dogs.[13] Because EIV and CIV are antigenically very similar, standard serologic tests cannot distinguish between infections caused by EIV or CIV. Accordingly, serologic data indicating low levels of CIV infection should not be given credibility in the absence of isolation of an influenza virus with the genetic signature of CIV.

The epidemiology of CIV in the United States has been unpredictable. Transmission of the virus among dogs readily occurs in group-housing situations such as animal shelters and boarding kennels, but the areas of the country where the virus is now enzootic are limited. The reasons for this defined geographic limitation are unknown. Outbreaks of CIV have occurred outside the enzootic areas of Florida, New York/Philadelphia, and Denver, but the virus has so far failed to become established in new areas (Dubovi, unpublished observations). CIV was isolated in San Diego (2006), Los Angeles (2007), Pittsburgh (2007), and Northern Virginia (2009), and dogs that tested positive in RT-PCR tests for CIV were detected in the Chicago area (2008), but none of these population centers have maintained the virus. CIV travels with dogs, and sporadic outbreaks have occurred in kennels that received rescue dogs taken from an enzootic area. Quarantine of the affected kennels stopped the spread of the virus. As with other mammalian-influenza virus interactions, there is no evidence for a true carrier state, so the maintenance of the virus depends on acute infections of susceptible populations. Although the virus is transmissible among dogs, it is not highly contagious perhaps because of the low amount of virus produced by the infected dogs (Dubovi, unpublished observation, 2007).[14]

H5N1

The emergence of a highly pathogenic avian influenza virus in 1996-1997 that was capable of causing significant respiratory disease in humans triggered an international surveillance program that tracked the movement of this family of viruses through Asia into Africa and Europe. In 2003, it was noted that this virus was capable of infecting felines, both domestic and exotics in zoo settings. The infections were initiated through the consumption of infected poultry. In October 2004, a 1-year-old dog in Thailand with severe respiratory signs died several days after ingesting a duck carcass from an area where the avian H5N1 virus was detected.[15] An influenza virus was isolated from tissues of the dog, and its genetic signature matched the H5N1 circulating in that area of Thailand.[16] The H5N1 virus clearly was capable of infecting mammals, but transmission from mammal to mammal was questionable.

Several studies were initiated to determine the response of dogs to infection by H5N1. In a limited transmission study using cats and dogs, no transmission could be detected in contact animals.[17] Infected animals had a low-grade fever for several days but were otherwise normal. In a second experimental infection, the exposed dogs again showed no clinical signs, but the virus could be detected by RT-PCR for several days.[18] Tests for influenza virus receptors in the respiratory tract of the dogs indicated that sialic acid–containing oligosaccharides existed on epithelial cells, and thus supported the possibility of influenza virus binding to sialic acid, leading to infection. Neither of the studies used the virus isolated from the fatal infection in Thailand, so a lack of clinical signs in the experimental infections could have been due to the use of a less-virulent isolate. At present, there is no evidence for transmission of H5N1 from an initially infected dog to a contact animal. Canine infections by H5N1 are most likely to be dead-end infections with little or no significance for the health of the canine population.

H3N2

In the summer of 2007, clinicians at 3 veterinary clinics in South Korea observed respiratory disease in individual dogs that eventually spread to several kennels. Nasal swabs from the affected dogs were inoculated into embryonated chicken eggs, and influenza virus was isolated from the cases.[19] Sequence analysis of the virus revealed it to be an avian-origin H3N2 virus. Comparisons with data in GenBank for all 8 gene segments revealed 95.5% to 98.9% homology to avian influenza viruses in East Asia. No contemporary avian isolates circulating in South Korea at the time of the canine infections were available for direct comparison with the canine isolates. It is not clear at present whether the virus involved in these cases was simply an avian virus with enhanced capability to infect dogs or a virus with a unique genetic signature enabling transmission in dogs, as with CIV. Virus isolated from the affected dogs was used to experimentally inoculate 10-week-old puppies, and the exposed animals showed typical signs of an acute respiratory infection within 2 days after infection.[20] Virus was recovered from nasal swabs, and sequence analysis showed that the recovered virus was identical to that used to initial the infection. The amount of virus shed in the experimentally infected animals significantly exceeded that found for the H3N8 CIV, suggesting that the H3N2 subtype is capable of more extensive replication in dogs. Although a dog-to-dog transmission study was also reported, the results were ambiguous because of the possibility that the in-contact dogs became infected by the original inoculum.

Serosurveys of the affected kennels showed a high prevalence for antibodies to H3N2 virus in the affected dogs, suggesting dog-to-dog transmission.[20] Additional serologic testing on companion animals not linked to dog farms or kennels showed H3N2 antibody prevalence rates of less than 5%.[21,22] Even though the prevalence is at a low level, the data do indicate that an H3N2 influenza virus is infecting dogs in South Korea. At this time there are no reports of H3N2 infections in other parts of the world.

H1N1

The detection of a novel H1N1 virus in clinical cases of respiratory disease in humans in early 2009 resulted in a worldwide effort to detect and control the spread of this agent. The detection of this virus in turkeys and swine raised interest in the monitoring for H1N1 in other mammalian species. At present, there are 2 undocumented reports of H1N1 infections in dogs. A report from China indicated that 2 of 52 sick dogs were positive for an H1N1 virus that was 99% homologous to the 2009 presumably human H1N1 virus.[23] A dog in New York State with a 2- to 3-day history of a respiratory infection tested positive for H1N1.[24] The dog's owner reported that he had also been tested positive for H1N1 earlier in the week. Given the intense surveillance for H1N1 infections, it is reasonable to conclude that this virus is not circulating in the dog population and that the rare infections arise from contact with infected owners. Infection of dogs with H1N1 in the areas that are enzootic to CIV does raise the possibility of coinfections generating recombinant viruses.

CLINICAL SIGNS AND INFECTION CHARACTERISTICS

At present, there are at least 7 viruses that are associated with acute respiratory disease in dogs (ARDD): influenza viruses, canine distemper virus, canine adenovirus 2, canine parainfluenza virus, canine respiratory coronavirus, canine herpesvirus, and most recently, canine pneumovirus.[25,26] The challenge in diagnosing influenza virus infections in dogs is similar to that for many respiratory pathogens in other species; the signs associated with the infection overlap with other agents. A clinician would find it hard, if not impossible, to distinguish the disease caused by an influenza virus infection from that caused by the other 6 viruses associated with ARDD. For CIV cases in the United States there is almost always a link to animal shelters, boarding kennels, or day care centers for dogs. The distinguishing feature, however, is the degree of morbidity within the facility. For most cases of ARDD, few dogs show signs because prior exposure and vaccination reduce the attack rate. For CIV, virtually all dogs are susceptible regardless of age, and attack rates of 60% to 80% are not unusual in group settings. The situation in South Korea with the H3N2 strain appears to be similar in that there was a high attack rate in dog farms and kennels, but low seroprevalence in companion animals.[21,22] Casual contact between dogs does not seem to be a high-risk factor, and this may relate to the relatively low amount of virus produced in dogs with CIV.

The signs associated with most influenza virus infections regardless of the H subtype are not pathognomonic for an influenza virus infection. The onset of clinical signs is usually rapid, with incubation periods in natural settings of 2 to 3 days being common. The detectable signs are somewhat related to the time from infection to the date of the examination. Common signs in most dogs are lethargy, anorexia, nasal discharge, sneezing, depression, ocular discharge, and cough, with coughing lasting up to 3 weeks postinfection. This range of clinical signs has been reproduced experimentally with both H3N8 CIV and the avian H3N2 virus.[14,20] Initially a nasal discharge may be clear, but it can quickly become mucopurulent. Many dogs show only a low-grade fever that may persist for 1 to 4 days. In uncomplicated cases a persistent, dry, and nonproductive cough develops, which may last for several weeks. Many dogs are diagnosed as having pneumonia, bronchopneumonia, or abnormal lung sounds. In natural settings, serious lung involvement is usually caused by the secondary bacteria, or mycoplasma infections that are enhanced with compromised lung defenses. In group settings, multiple viral pathogens may be circulating, which further complicates the identity of a causative agent (Dubovi, unpublished observation, 2009).[26] The mortality rate directly as a result of influenza virus infections is difficult to determine, given the negative effect of other respiratory agents.

In several experimental models, the basic pathophysiology of the influenza virus infections was reproduced in the apparent absence of secondary agents.[14,19,20,27,28] After challenge, clinical signs could be detected as early as 1 day postinfection, with 2 days being more common. As with natural infections, early signs were ocular discharge, nasal discharge, and lethargy accompanied by a low-grade fever. The peak of the virus shed is 2 to 4 days postinfection, with the viable virus as determined by virus isolation becoming undetectable by day 7 postinfection. The detection of a viral signal from a nasal swab can be extended to 10 days postinfection in rare cases with the use of RT-PCR. The immune response to influenza virus infections as determined by hemagglutination inhibition (HI) titers is rapid, with detectable responses by 7 days postinfection.[14,20] Both experimental infections and field data indicate that the infected dogs do not shed virus beyond 10 days postinfection. Dogs that continue to cough beyond this period are not at risk for transmitting the virus.

The extent of the pathologic lesions produced by influenza virus infections is affected by the host and the strain of the virus. In an experimental study using 3 CIV strains, Deshpande and colleagues[14] showed that 2 of the 3 challenge strains gave higher shedding titers than the third virus, and 1 of the 3 strains induced more severe clinical signs. All challenge data for the avian-origin H3N2 have been done with the same virus, so no viral comparisons are available.[20,27] As one could expect with a respiratory pathogen, the early lesions in the upper respiratory tract are consistent with tracheitis and bronchitis with some extension to the bronchioles. There are areas of epithelial cell necrosis, loss of cuboidal glandular cells, and infiltration of the propria-submucosa by mixtures of inflammatory cells. As a result, the normal defense of the respiratory tract provided by the ciliated epithelial cells is severely compromised. The effect of the virus infection on the lower respiratory tract can be highly variable, and the lesions noted are more severe in the later stages of the infection. On day 3 postinfection, there were numerous petechial hemorrhages in most lobes of the lung.[14] At later times in the infection, consolidated areas of the lung could be seen, which coincided with an increase in clinical signs. Histopathological lesions consisted of peribronchiolar and perivascular infiltration of lymphocytes and plasma cells (tracheobronchitis and bronchiolitis), diffuse thickening of alveolar septa by infiltrates of inflammatory cells, and infiltration of the alveoli by neutrophils and macrophages (alveolitis).[14,27,28] The reported lesions were in animals that tested negative for other pathogens, which indicates that influenza virus alone is able to cause significant pathologic changes.

DIAGNOSTICS

A successful laboratory diagnosis of canine respiratory infections greatly depends on the timing of the collection of specimens for agent detection tests. As noted for influenza virus infections (and most other viral pathogens of the respiratory tract), the period for which the virus exists in the infected animal is relatively short. As indicated earlier, the incubation period for influenza virus is about 2 days with maximum virus shed in the 2- to 4-day period. The experimental data clearly show that infectious virus is no longer detectable by 7 days postinfection.[14,20] For individual dogs, it would be unusual for owners to seek veterinary care in less than 4 days after infection and 2 days after onset of clinical signs. Sampling to detect the virus must be done at first contact with the patient. Waiting for several days to obtain a response to antibiotic treatment will lead to negative test results even though the animal may have been infected.

The current test of choice to detect influenza virus is RT-PCR with the target being the matrix gene. Tests have been validated to detect virtually any H subtype of influenza virus. The initial determination is whether any type of influenza virus is involved in the clinical event. If the initial test result is positive, then the subtype of influenza virus can be determined by ancillary tests. In this manner any of the various influenza viruses identified in dogs can be detected. Samples of choice are nasal swabs, either cotton or Dacron. Because RT-PCR does not depend on viability for a successful test, the transport medium is not critical, but it should not be a bacterial transport medium that has not been validated for RT-PCR. A few drops of saline to keep the swab moist is more than adequate.

Virus isolations can be done using either Madin-Darby canine kidney (MDCK) cells or embryonated chicken eggs. Both procedures have proven successful in isolating the virus, but some samples yield virus with one procedure but not the other (Dubovi, unpublished observation). The basis for this observation is unknown. For egg inoculation, the sample should be blind passed at least once because the H3-subtype viruses give poor yields in eggs.

Antigen-capture enzyme-linked immunosorbent assay (ELISA) tests are not of great value when assessing the infection status of a single dog. The reasons for this are timing and the low level of virus produced by the infected dogs. At best, the tests are 50% sensitive and should be used only in multiple-dog outbreaks where the timing factor is discounted by sampling of multiple dogs at various stages of infection. Its use in this context is simply to define the presence of virus in a group-housing situation, and in that context, the tests can have significant value.

Testing to detect previous exposure to influenza viruses in dogs has been problematic. The most sensitive test historically was the HI test, but to use this test to screen for any exposure, one had to use 16 different viruses to cover all influenza virus H subtypes. For HI testing one has to be aware of nonspecific reactions in the testing that can lead to false positives. An agar-gel immunodiffusion test using the nucleoprotein (NP) as an antigen successfully detects any influenza virus infection in poultry, but it lacks sensitivity in mammalian systems. ELISA tests using the same NP antigen are now in use at present for avian samples and were used for dogs in Korea.

For CIV in the United States, the HI test is the standard test used for serologic determinations. The test has high sensitivity because it can detect antibody responses in dogs in as early as 7 days postinfection.[14] In the absence of other H subtypes of influenza virus in circulation, it is the test of choice. In clinical cases where the dog has shown clinical signs for more than 5 days, agent detection tests are rarely successful, so serology should be used to define an influenza virus infection. Acute and convalescent sampling can be done, but with the low prevalence of infection in the United States, a single sample collected more than 7 days after onset of signs is highly useful in defining exposure.

TREATMENT AND PREVENTION

As indicated earlier, respiratory disease in dogs may be caused by any 1 of 7 different viruses, several different bacterial species, and at least 1 species of mycoplasma. For the academic, it is important to know which agents are involved in order to develop prevention strategies, but for the clinician, knowing which virus initiated the infection may be of little value. Treatment of the individual animal from a single-pet household is largely the same regardless of the agent involved; treatment involves coverage with a broad-spectrum antibiotic to prevent or treat a bacterial or mycoplasma-enhanced pneumonia. For the individual dog, the cost to determine the causative agent may be difficult to justify to the owner if the treatment is unaffected by the outcome. For kennel situations, it is important to know the precipitating agent because this may dictate the manner in which the animals are managed and whether movement restrictions are in order.

When discussing influenza virus, the issue of antiviral drugs invariably arises. To be effective, these drugs need to be administered very early in the infection cycle. Again for the individual dog, treatment would most likely begin after the effective period had been passed. For kennels, there might be reasons to consider these drugs, but at present there are no data on the effectiveness of these drugs in treating influenza virus in dogs. Unfounded use of the drugs is simply an invitation for the selection of drug-resistant variants.

At present, there is a vaccine licensed by the US Department of Agriculture for CIV in the United States. A vaccine was also developed for the avian-origin H3N2 in Korea, but its commercial distribution is unclear. In both instances, the vaccines are killed adjuvanted products.[29,30] Challenge studies testing both products reported decreases in virus shedding and lung pathology compared with the nonvaccinated challenge group. As expected, the vaccines did not prevent infection, a finding that is consistent with virtually all killed influenza-virus products in any species. There are no data on the duration of immunity, but yearly vaccinations are recommended. In those settings where there is a defined risk for influenza virus infections, these vaccines would be appropriate to be recommended with the same justification as traditional kennel cough vaccines.

SUMMARY

In cases of respiratory disease in canines, influenza viruses should be on the list of agents that can infect dogs and cause clinical disease. The presence of specific subtypes of influenza virus capable of being transmitted from dog to dog is at present geographically limited to the United States and Korea. Other subtypes have been detected in dogs, but transmission to other dogs has not occurred. As surveillance intensifies to meet the concerns of the human population with respect to pandemic influenza viruses, more cases of influenza virus in dogs are certain to be detected. Each infection offers an opportunity for a unique variant to emerge and continue the evolution of influenza virus as a species-crossing pathogen.

REFERENCES

1. Nikitin T, Cohen D, Todd JD, et al. Epidemiological studies of A/Hong Kong/68 virus infection in dogs. Bull Wld Hlth Org 1972;47:471–9.
2. Kilbourne ED, Kehoe JM. Demonstration of antibodies to both hemagglutinin and neuraminidase antigens of H3H2 influenza A virus in domestic dogs. Intervirology 1975-76;6:315–8.
3. Crawford PC, Dubovi EJ, Castleman WL, et al. Transmission of equine influenza virus to dogs. Science 2005;310:482–5.
4. Payungporn S, Crawford PC, Kouo TS, et al. Isolation and characterization of influenza A subtype H3N8 viruses from dogs with respiratory disease in Florida. Emerg Infect Dis 2008;14:902–8.
5. Dubovi EJ, Njaa BL. Canine influenza. Vet Clin Small Anim 2008;38:827–35.
6. Beeler E. Influenza in dogs and cats. Vet Clin Small Anim 2009;39:251–64.
7. Harder TC, Vahlenkamp TW. Influenza virus infections in dogs and cats. Vet Immunol Immunopath 2010;134:54–60.
8. Gibbs EP, Anderson TC. Equine and canine influenza: a review of current events. Anim Health Res Rev 2010;29:1–9.
9. Yoon KJ, Cooper VL, Schwartz KJ, et al. Influenza virus infection in racing greyhounds. Emerg Infect Dis 2005;11:1974–5.
10. Jirjis FF, Deshpande MS, Tubbs AL, et al. Transmission of canine influenza virus (H3N8) among susceptible dogs. Vet Microbiol 2010;144(3–4):303–9.
11. Daly JM, Blunden AS, MacRae S, et al. Transmission of equine influenza virus to English foxhounds. Emerg Infect Dis 2008;14:461–4.
12. Kirkland P, Finlaison DS, Crispe E, et al. Influenza virus transmission from horses to dogs: Australia. Emerg Infect Dis 2010;16:699–702.

13. Tamanaka T, Nemoto M, Tsujimura K, et al. Interspecies transmission of equine influenza virus (H3N8) to dogs by close contact with experimentally infected horses. Vet Microbiol 2009;39:351–5.
14. Deshpande MS, Abdelmagid O, Tubbs A, et al. Experimental reproduction of canine influenza virus H3N8 infection in young puppies. Vet Therapeutics 2009; 10:29–39.
15. Songserm T, Amonsin A, Jam-on R, et al. Fatal avian influenza A H5N1 in a dog. Emerg Infect Dis 2006;12:1744–6.
16. Amonsin A, Songserm T, Chutinimitkul S, et al. Genetic analysis of influenza A virus (H5N1) derived from domestic cat and dog in Thailand. Arch Virol 2007; 152:1925–33.
17. Giese M, Harder TC, Teifke JP, et al. Experimental infection and natural contact exposure of dogs with avian influenza virus (H5N1). Emerg Infect Dis 2008;14: 308–10.
18. Maas R, Tacken M, Ruuls L, et al. Avian influenza (H5N1) susceptibility and receptors in dogs. Emerg Infect Dis 2007;13:1219–21.
19. Song D, Kang B, Lee C, et al. Transmission of avian influenza virus (H3N2) to dogs. Emerg Infect Dis 2008;14:741–6.
20. Song D, Lee C, Kang B, et al. Experimental infection of dogs with avian-origin canine influenza A virus (H3N2). Emerg Infect Dis 2009;15:56–8.
21. Lee C, Song D, Kang B, et al. A serological survey of avian origin canine H3N2 influenza virus in dogs in Korea. Vet Microbiol 2009;137:359–62.
22. An DJ, Jeoung HY, Jeong W, et al. A serological survey of canine respiratory coronavirus and canine influenza virus in Korean dogs. J Vet Med Sci 2010. [Epub ahead of print].
23. Promed posting: Archive Number 20091128.4079. Published date 28 November 2009 [online].
24. Promed posting: Archive Number 20091222.4305. Published date 22 December 2009 [online].
25. Erles K, Dubovi EJ, Brooks HW, et al. Longitudinal study of viruses associated with canine infectious respiratory disease. J Clin Microbiol 2004;42:4524–9.
26. Renshaw RR, Zylich NC, Laverack MA, et al. Pneumovirus in dogs acutely with acute respiratory disease. Emerg Infect Dis 2010;16:993–5.
27. Jung K, Lee CS, Kang BK, et al. Pathology in dogs with experimental canine H3N2 influenza virus infection. Res Vet Sci 2010,88:523–7.
28. Castleman WL, Powe JR, Crawford PC, et al. Canine H3N8 influenza virus infection in dogs and mice. Vet Pathol 2010;47:507–17.
29. Deshpande MS, Jirjis FF, Tubbs AL, et al. Evaluation of the efficacy of a canine influenza virus (H3N8) vaccine in dogs following experimental challenge. Vet Therapeutics 2009;10:103–12.
30. Lee C, Jung K, Oh J, et al. Protective efficacy and immunogenicity of an inactivated avian-origin H3N2 canine influenza vaccine in dogs challenged with the virulent virus. Vet Microbiol 2010;143:184–8.

Feline Bartonellosis

Lynn Guptill, DVM, PhD

KEYWORDS

• *Bartonella* • Cat • Feline • Bartonellosis
• Vector • Flea • Bacteremia

CAUSE

Bartonella are small, fastidious, vector-transmitted gram-negative bacteria in the family Bartonellaceae of the α-2 subgroup of the Proteobacteria.[1] These bacteria are highly adapted to mammalian reservoir hosts, in which a long-term asymptomatic bacteremia often occurs. The type species is *B bacilliformis*, an intracellular parasite of human erythrocytes and endothelial cells that causes severe hemolytic anemia and cutaneous angioproliferative lesions in human beings. It is endemic to some countries in South America and is transmitted among human beings by *Lutzomyia* sp sand-flies.[1,2] In addition to the type species, the *Bartonella* species includes organisms that originally comprised the genera *Rochalimaea* and *Grahamella*.[1,3] The *Bartonellas* are phylogenetically close to the *Rickettsiae* and bacteria of the species *Brucella*, *Agrobacterium*, and *Afipia*.[4-6] At least 22 species of *Bartonella* are officially named, and numerous other species are pending formal naming. Approximately 14 *Bartonella* species are considered zoonotic, and of these zoonotic species, several are trans-mitted to human beings via companion animals, including some transmitted by cats.

The primary zoonotic *Bartonella* species associated with cats is *B henselae*, which causes bacteremia in healthy cats, and has been detected by polymerase chain reac-tion (PCR) in tissues of numerous other mammalian species, including dogs, seals, whales, horses, and wild felids.[7-12] *B henselae* causes cat scratch disease (CSD), bacillary angiomatosis, bacillary peliosis, relapsing fever with bacteremia, meningitis, encephalitis, neuroretinitis, endocarditis, and multiple additional clinical entities in human beings.[13-17] *B clarridgeiae* causes bacteremia in healthy cats,[18,19] and was serologically associated with a CSD-like condition in 2 people.[20,21] It was also asso-ciated with aortic valve endocarditis in a dog,[22] and was detected by PCR in the liver of a dog with hepatopathy.[12] *B koehlerae*[23] was isolated from 4 healthy cats, and has been associated with human endocarditis.[24] *B koehlerae* did not cause clinical signs in cats inoculated experimentally, but was associated with endocarditis in a dog.[25,26] It has not been established that *B quintana* is zoonotic. *B quintana* caused trench fever in World War I and is now known to cause endocarditis, bacillary angiomatosis,

Department of Veterinary Clinical Sciences, Purdue University, 625 Harrison Street, West Lafayette, IN 47907, USA
E-mail address: guptillc@purdue.edu

Vet Clin Small Anim 40 (2010) 1073–1090
doi:10.1016/j.cvsm.2010.07.009   vetsmall.theclinics.com
0195-5616/10/$ – see front matter © 2010 Elsevier Inc. All rights reserved.

bacillary peliosis, and chronic lymphadenomegaly in people. Human beings are considered the reservoir host for *B quintana*, and it is transmitted among human beings by the human body louse.[27,28] *B quintana* has been identified in tissues of domestic cats and other animals, but whether *B quintana* should be considered zoonotic is not yet defined.[29,30] *Candidatus* B rochalimae was associated with febrile disease in one human being, and has been detected in wild foxes.[31,32] This organism was also detected in a dog with endocarditis.[33] Cats inoculated experimentally with *candidatus* B rochalimae exhibited no clinical signs of illness.[34] Dogs and foxes are considered likely reservoir hosts for *candidatus* B rochalimae.

This article focuses on feline bartonellosis, in particular on *B henselae*, as it is the feline-associated *Bartonella* for which the most information is known. *B henselae* is an important zoonotic agent with the cat as the primary mammalian reservoir.

EPIDEMIOLOGY

Feline *B henselae* infection was first reported in 1992.[35] Since then, natural infection of cats with 5 *Bartonella* species (*B henselae*, *B clarridgeiae*, *B koehlerae*, *B quintana*, and *B bovis* [formerly *B weissii*])[21,23,30,36–38] has been reported, although feline infections with species other than *B henselae* or *B clarridgeiae* are rarely reported.[21,23,36,38] Seroepidemiologic studies of cats indicate that exposure to *Bartonella* species, most frequently *B henselae*, occurs worldwide. Seroprevalence is greatest in warm, humid climates, particularly in older cats, feral cats, and cats infested with fleas.[39–44] *B henselae* bacteremia occurs in approximately 5% to 40% of cats in the United States on average, also with a higher prevalence in warmer, more humid regions with high flea prevalence.[19,41,45] In some cat colonies, *Bartonella* seroprevalence is as high as 90%.[44] In one study, most cats belonging to people with CSD had *B henselae* bacteremia.[46] Approximately 10% of cats with *Bartonella* bacteremia in the United States were infected with *B clarridgeiae*. Approximately 30% of cats in studies in France and in the Philippines with *Bartonella* bacteremia were infected with *B clarridgeiae*.[43,47,48] *B koehlerae* was isolated from 2 cats from one household in California, 1 cat in France and 1 cat in Israel and *B bovis* (formerly *B weissii*) was isolated from a cat in Utah and one in Illinois.[23,24,38,49] Domestic cats are considered the primary mammalian reservoir and vector for human infections with *B henselae*. Cats may be the reservoir for *B clarridgeiae*, and cattle are the reservoir for *B bovis*. The reservoir for *B koehlerae* is believed to be the cat. Human beings are considered the primary reservoir for *B quintana*.

Wild felids are also exposed to *Bartonella* infection. Eighteen percent of panthers in Florida, 28% of mountain lions in Texas, 30% to 53% of free-ranging and captive wild felids in California, 17% of African lions, and 31% of African cheetahs had serum antibodies to *B henselae*.[50–52] *Bartonella* species were also identified by culture or PCR testing in wild African lions and cheetahs.

B henselae are genetically diverse. There are 2 primary 16S rRNA types of *B henselae*, and at least 2 subgroups within each type.[53] Coinfection of cats with *B henselae* 16S rRNA types I and II, and with *B henselae* and *B clarridgeiae* is reported.[18,54,55] There are regional differences in prevalence of infection of cats with different rRNA types of *B henselae*.[42,43,47,54] Other molecular methods also show remarkable molecular diversity among *Bartonella* isolates.[56–65] There is evidence of genomic variation in *B henselae* during the course of infection in cats.[56–64] Such variation likely enhances the ability of *B henselae* to persist in infected cats for prolonged periods. Genetic variation makes vaccine development difficult, although it is useful in epidemiologic studies, and may also be useful in furthering the understanding of the pathogenicity of various *Bartonella* isolates.[65–67]

PATHOGENESIS

B henselae is naturally transmitted among cats by cat fleas (*Ctenocephalides felis felis*). *B henselae* was transmitted among cats by transferring fleas fed on infected cats to specific pathogen-free cats, and by intradermal inoculation of excrement from infected fleas.[68,69] *B henselae* survives for at least 3 days in flea feces, suggesting that flea feces are an important source of environmental contamination.[70] Cats did not become infected with *B henselae* when fed on by *Bartonella*-infected fleas enclosed in capsules that prevented contamination of cats with flea excrement.[69] This finding suggests that transmission does not occur via flea saliva. It has been suggested that ticks may have a role in transmission, as *Bartonella* spp are found in some questing ticks.[14,71–76] There is evidence of transstadial infection of *Ixodes ricinus* ticks with *B henselae*, and *B henselae* was detected in the saliva of infected ticks.[77] *Bartonella* species have also been detected in biting flies.[78] However, detection of *Bartonella* in arthropod vectors found feeding on vertebrate hosts infected with *Bartonella* species does not indicate that the arthropods are competent vectors, and there is no published evidence that ticks or biting flies can serve as biologic vectors for *Bartonella* species.[79]

In laboratory studies cats were experimentally infected with *B henselae* through intravenous or intramuscular[55] inoculation with infected cat blood, by intravenous, subcutaneous, intradermal, or oral inoculation with laboratory-grown bacteria, and via infestation with *Bartonella*-infected fleas or intradermal inoculation of *Bartonella*-infected flea feces.[68,69,80] *B henselae* transmission did not occur when infected cats cohabited with uninfected cats in a flea-free environment,[81,82] indicating that transmission among cats does not occur directly through cat bites, scratches, grooming, or sharing of food dishes and litter boxes when fleas are absent. Transmission did not occur when cats were inoculated intramuscularly with urine of bacteremic cats.[83] There was no transmission between flea-free *B henselae*-bacteremic female cats and uninfected males during mating, nor was there transplacental or transmammary transmission to kittens.[82,84]

Feline bacteremia with *B henselae* is commonly chronic and recurrent. Experimentally infected cats in arthropod-free environments maintained relapsing *B henselae* or *B clarridgeiae* bacteremia for as long as 454 days, with relapses of bacteremia occurring at irregular intervals of between 1 and 4.5 months.[55,85] Relapsing bacteremia was reported in naturally infected cats for 3 years; however, this finding may have represented reinfection over time as a result of re-exposure to infected fleas.[46] A recent report documents persistent relapsing bacteremia in cats as a result of reinfection of cats with different strains of *B henselae* over time.[86]

Measured increases in interleukin-4 mRNA and serum antibody titers following the peak of bacteremia occurred concurrent with a decrease in bacteremia to low or undetectable levels in one study.[87] However, the effectiveness of antibodies in clearing bacteremia is not certain. In another study, kittens that did not produce measurable anti-*Bartonella* IgM or IgG antibodies had the same course of bacteremia as did kittens that produced high titers of anti-*Bartonella* antibodies.[85] Results of a recent study suggest that cell-mediated immunity is important in reducing the level of bacteremia in experimentally infected cats.[88] Cats maintained normal CD4 and CD8 lymphocyte numbers and ratios in one experimental study, whereas in another study some experimentally infected cats had transiently decreased CD4 lymphocyte numbers.[81,88]

Cats seem to be protected from reinfection with homologous strains of *B henselae*, but not always against heterologous challenge. Cats previously infected with *B henselae* 16S rRNA type II were not protected from infection with *B henselae* 16S rRNA type I,[89] but were protected against homologous challenge. Cats infected with *B henselae* type I or II were susceptible to challenge infection with *B clarridgeiae*, and cats infected with *B koehlerae* or *B clarridgeiae* were susceptible to challenge infection with *B henselae* type I or type II. In contrast, cats infected with *B henselae* type I were partially or completely protected against challenge infection with *B henselae* type II.[90] The level of bacteremia and degree of susceptibility to reinfection following challenge inoculation varies with strain, as well as with species, of *Bartonella*.

The localization of *Bartonella* in cats has not been completely determined. *Bartonella* are generally intracellular bacteria, and *B henselae* have been detected within erythrocytes of naturally infected cats.[91] *Bartonella* may also be located intracellularly in vascular endothelial cells of infected cats as has been suggested for rats infected with *B tribocorum*.[92] Extracellular *B henselae* are also detected in blood and other tissues of infected cats.[93]

CLINICAL FINDINGS
Experimental Studies

Most cats experimentally infected with *Bartonella* exhibited no clinical signs. Clinical signs that did occur were generally mild, and varied with the strain of *B henselae* used for inoculation.[55,81,94] Cats inoculated intradermally developed areas of induration and/or abscess at inoculation sites between approximately 2 and 21 days after inoculation.[55,81,83,95] Pure cultures of *B henselae* were obtained from these lesions in some cats.[81] Other transient clinical findings included generalized or localized peripheral lymphadenomegaly that persisted for approximately 6 weeks after inoculation, and short periods of fever (>103°F; 39.4°C) during the first 48 to 96 hours after inoculation and again for 24 to 48 hours at approximately 2 weeks after inoculation. Some cats were lethargic and anorexic when febrile. Mild neurologic signs (nystagmus, transient whole body tremors, transient decreased or exaggerated responses to external stimuli, transient, mild behavior changes) and epaxial muscle pain were also reported in some cats.[81,83,94,96] In one cat infected experimentally via flea infestation, severe cardiac disease resulted and the cat was euthanatized.[80] Reproductive failure occurred in some cats.[84] There were no reported clinical signs in cats experimentally infected with *B koehlerae* or *candidatus* B rochalimae.[25,34]

Clinicopathologic and histopathologic findings (complete blood counts, serum biochemical tests, and urine analysis) were normal in most experimentally infected cats.[55,81,83,94,96] A few cats had transient mild anemia early in the course of infection, and some had persistent eosinophilia.[55] Mature neutrophilia occurred in some cats during periods of skin inflammation.[81] Cats had hyperplasia of lymphoid organs, small foci of lymphocytic, pyogranulomatous, or neutrophilic inflammation in multiple tissues (lung, liver, spleen, kidney, heart), and small foci of necrosis in the liver or spleen.[55,81]

Natural Infection

Clinical signs are uncommon in naturally infected cats. No clinical signs were reported in 65 naturally infected cats.[54] One cat with uveitis was serologically positive for *B henselae* infection with evidence of ocular production of anti-*Bartonella* IgG antibodies.[97] Seven (14%) of 49 animals in a convenience sample of cats with uveitis had evidence of ocular production of anti-*Bartonella* IgG antibodies.[98] In another study, healthy cats were more likely to be seropositive for *Bartonella* than were cats with uveitis.[99]

Bartonella was associated with endocarditis in 3 naturally infected cats.[100,101] B henselae DNA was detected in the aortic valves of these cats with endocarditis, and occasional silver-stained coccoid structures were seen in endothelial cells of the myocardium. Whether members of the genus Bartonella contribute to previously described instances of argyrophilic bacteria in lymph nodes of cats with persistent lymphadenomegaly is unknown.[102] Bartonella DNA was not found in tissues of 14 cats with plasmacytic pododermatitis, or 26 cats with peliosis hepatis, and immunohistochemical staining was negative for Bartonella in these cats.[103,104]

A potential causative role of Bartonella spp in chronic diseases of cats has been proposed because Bartonella bacteremia in cats is often prolonged. However, contribution of Bartonella infections to development of chronic illnesses of cats has not been verified. Findings of a study in Japan[105] suggested that cats seropositive for B henselae and feline immunodeficiency virus (FIV) were more likely to have gingivitis or lymphadenomegaly than were cats seropositive for either agent alone. Results of a Swiss study[106] suggested possible associations between B henselae seropositivity and stomatitis and various urinary tract disorders. However, the usefulness of serology for establishing Bartonella infection seems to be limited, and conclusions drawn from studies that rely on serologic methods for diagnosis of Bartonella infection should be interpreted with caution (see next section on diagnosis).

Clinical conditions proposed as attributable to feline bartonellosis may also result from other causes, and it is difficult to determine in which cats Bartonella infection does cause clinical signs. Case-control studies evaluating naturally infected cats have not proved an association of Bartonella with anemia, gingivostomatitis, neurologic conditions, or uveitis. In some of these studies, animals seropositive for Bartonella were less likely to be affected by the clinical condition studied than were serologically negative animals.[99,107–110] These results underscore the difficulty in establishing causal associations between clinical conditions and a pathogen like Bartonella that has a high prevalence in the reservoir host population. The prevalence of Bartonella DNA in the blood of febrile cats was nearly statistically significantly greater ($P = 0.057$) than the prevalence of Bartonella DNA in the blood of afebrile cats.[111] Afebrile control cats in that study were significantly more likely to be seropositive for Bartonella than were febrile cats, again highlighting the difficulty in interpreting serologic tests for Bartonella in cats, and indicating that serologic testing alone is not indicated for evaluation of ill cats. There was no support for Bartonella as a cause of chronic rhinosinusitis in cats in a study comparing cats with rhinosinusitis, cats with other nasal disease, cats with other systemic illnesses, and healthy control cats, although the power of this study to detect a difference among groups was low.[112] Another study[113] reported no association between Bartonella seropositivity and results of feline pancreatic lipase immunoreactivity tests, suggesting that serologic testing for Bartonella is not indicated for cats with pancreatitis.

Because of the high prevalence of Bartonella exposure in the domestic cat population, additional extensive, carefully controlled epidemiologic investigations are needed to determine whether particular clinical conditions are truly associated with B henselae infections in cats. The likelihood that some clinical conditions have multiple causes must also be considered, particularly in cats with exposure to arthropod vectors.

DIAGNOSIS

Diagnosis of Bartonella infection is not straightforward. Clinical signs, when present, are transient and variable, and determining which sick animals are most likely to have Bartonella infection is difficult. Because bartonellosis is zoonotic, veterinarians may be asked to test healthy pets belonging to clients with *Bartonella*-related illnesses, or to screen healthy cats that are being considered as pets for immunocompromised people (see section on public health).

Cytology

Detecting *B henselae* in erythrocytes of infected cats has not been effective for diagnosis using conventional staining methods. Intraerythrocytic *B clarridgeiae* and *B koehlerae* were documented in naturally infected cats using fluorescent antibody detection methods.[49,91] In addition, extracellular *B henselae* have been documented in peripheral blood and other tissues of infected cats using immunocytochemical and immunohistochemical methods.[93]

Serology

Serologic testing alone as a diagnostic tool is problematic in that false-positive test results seem to be common regardless of the assay used. Serology is probably best used in conjunction with blood culture or PCR testing. Serum IgG antibodies persist in experimentally infected animals for prolonged periods, and how long antibodies persist following clearance of an infection is unknown. It remains difficult to document clearance of *Bartonella* infection, because of the relapsing nature of feline bacteremia, and relative insensitivity of culture and molecular methods to detect low levels of bacteremia. False-negative results are less common; 5% to 12% of cats with *B henselae* bacteremia are seronegative.[54,114]

Immunofluorescent antibody (IFA), enzyme immunoassay (EIA) and Western blot tests are available. Infections with some strains or species of *Bartonella* may be missed using any serologic method, depending on the antigen preparations used.[115] Positive predictive values of IFA and EIA tests for anti-*B henselae* serum IgG antibodies for bacteremia in cats are 39% to 46%. The usefulness of a negative serologic test is greater, as the negative predictive values for these tests in cats are high, at 89% to 97%.[42,54,114] The diagnostic accuracy of Western blot tests has not been so extensively investigated. Results of one study showed no differences in Western blot patterns for cats evaluated over the course of infection, whereas in another study, antibodies of sera of infected cats reacted with an increasing number of bands of polyacrylamide gel-separated antigens over time.[55,116] Another study reported that the positive predictive value of a Western blot test for presence of *B henselae* DNA in cat blood was only 18.8%.[110]

Bacterial Isolation

A positive blood culture or culture of other tissue is the most reliable test for definitive diagnosis of active *Bartonella* infection. Because of the relapsing nature of feline *Bartonella* bacteremia, a single blood culture is not a sensitive diagnostic tool for bacteremia, and multiple blood cultures may be necessary.[117]

Blood for culture should be obtained using sterile technique and the blood placed in ethylenediamine tetraacetic acid (EDTA)-containing tubes or lysis centrifugation blood culture tubes (Isolator tubes, Wampole, Cranbury, NJ, USA). If blood is collected into EDTA tubes the blood should be chilled or frozen for transport to the laboratory. Blood should be sent to laboratories familiar with the culture of these fastidious organisms. Enriched media and special culture conditions are necessary for successful isolation of *Bartonella*, and incubation times may be prolonged. Although likely not necessary for blood culture for most cats suspected of having bartonellosis, the recent development of a novel pre-enrichment medium for *Bartonella* culture may make blood culture a more sensitive diagnostic tool.[118] The use of this newer diagnostic protocol may enhance detection of *Bartonella* species in nonreservoir hosts. The importance of strict sterile technique when collecting blood samples for culture cannot be overemphasized, as enriched media are routinely used for *Bartonella* culture. Even a small amount of contamination may result in overgrowth with less fastidious bacteria, or conversely, it is conceivable that residual flea excrement at the site of venipuncture may result in a positive *Bartonella* culture with the use of enriched media. Laboratories should be contacted for specific instructions for sample collection and submission.

Nucleic Acid Detection

Standard PCR testing for *Bartonella* DNA in blood may be no more sensitive than blood culture for detection of active *Bartonella* infection, and detecting DNA does not always equate to detection of living organisms. Real-time PCR improves diagnostic sensitivity. The primer pairs used in PCR testing have a marked influence on the sensitivity of PCR assays.[119] An advantage of PCR testing is that the results are often available more quickly than those of blood culture. The products of PCR reactions may be sequenced and species and/or strain of *Bartonella* therefore identified, making rapid differentiation of pathogenic *Bartonella* species possible.[120] Samples for PCR testing should be obtained using strict sterile technique, and care must be taken in collection and processing to avoid sample contamination (and false-positive results) or DNA degradation (and false-negative results). Contact individual laboratories for collection and submission guidelines.

Coinfection

Pets may be coinfected with multiple pathogens, for example, cats may be coinfected with other vector-borne pathogens such as hemotrophic *Mycoplasmas* or rickettsial pathogens.[108,121] Cats may also be coinfected with feline leukemia virus or FIV and *Bartonella* species. Such coinfections make attributing clinical signs of disease to infection with a particular organism difficult, and also have important implications for therapy.

TREATMENT

Documenting clearance of feline *Bartonella* infections through antibiotic treatment is difficult because of the relapsing nature of the bacteremia. Treatment of *Bartonella* infections seems to require long-term (at least 4–6 weeks) antibiotic administration. No regimen of antibiotic treatment has been proved effective for definitively eliminating *Bartonella* infections in cats.[45,95,122] Enrofloxacin (3.5–11.4 mg/kg given by mouth every 12 hours) treatment for 28 days appeared to clear *B henselae* or *B clarridgeiae* infection in 5 of 7 treated cats that were monitored for 12 weeks after treatment.[45] However, enrofloxacin causes retinal degeneration and blindness in some cats when administered at more than 5 mg/kg/d, and use of a higher dose is contraindicated.[123] Results of a recent study showed good in vitro efficacy of pradofloxacin against *B henselae*.[124] However, another report documented naturally occurring fluoroquinolone resistance in *Bartonella* isolates, and it was recommended that no fluoroquinolones be used to treat any *Bartonella*-related clinical condition in human beings.[125] Doxycycline (6.9–12.8 mg/kg by mouth every 12 hours) appeared to clear *B henselae* or *B clarridgeiae* infection in one of 6 cats treated for 2 weeks; doxycycline (4–10.4 mg/kg by mouth every 12 hours) for 4 weeks appeared to clear infection in one of 2 cats[45]; and doxycycline (50 mg/cat by mouth every 12 hours for 1 week) appeared to clear infection in 4 of 8 cats.[95] The higher doses of doxycycline may be more likely to be effective for treating feline *Bartonella* infections. Antibiotics tested in other studies (erythromycin, amoxicillin, amoxicillin/clavulanic acid, tetracycline hydrochloride) decreased the level of bacteremia in treated cats. However, the cats were not followed for a prolonged period after treatment. In another study, antibiotic treatment could not be deemed successful compared with no treatment because untreated cats became blood culture negative after the same length of time as did cats that were treated.[122] Rifampin used in combination with doxycycline has been recommended, but data regarding efficacy of this combination in cats have not been published. Rifampin should not be used alone, because resistance develops quickly.[126]

Azithromycin has been widely used to treat feline *Bartonella* infections, but there are no data from controlled studies to support this practice. Azithromycin was shown in a controlled clinical trial to have some efficacy for limiting lymph node enlargement in people with CSD, and since has been widely adopted as a treatment of cats.[127] Macrolide-resistant strains of *Bartonella* are reported, and concern was stated in one publication that these may arise as a result of animals being treated with macrolide antibiotics.[128] Recent in vitro data suggest that the efficacy of azithromycin against *Bartonella* may be limited, and resistance to azithromycin arises in vitro as well.[124] Also, azithromycin seems to have important immunomodulatory and antiinflammatory properties in addition to its broad antimicrobial spectrum.[129-132] Another macrolide, erythromycin, markedly diminished endothelial cell proliferation induced by *B quintana* in an in vitro model, and this effect was not related to the bacteriostatic effects of the drug.[133] It is therefore difficult to determine whether reports of beneficial effects after azithromycin treatment of cats are solely a result of anti-*Bartonella* activity or instead are a result of the other properties of azithromycin, of the antimicrobial action of azithromycin on other bacteria, or of a combination of all of these. These data suggest that azithromycin is not the best first choice for treating feline bartonellosis.

People with *Bartonella* infections causing bacillary angiomatosis or peliosis, or endocarditis, are treated with a variety of antibiotics, including trimethoprim-sulfamethoxazole, doxycycline, erythromycin, ciprofloxacin, rifampin, gentamicin, clarithromycin, and azithromycin.[134] Rifampin resistance was readily induced in *B quintana*, and it is recommended that people with *Bartonella* infections never be treated with rifampin alone.[126] Gentamicin resistance was induced in *B henselae* only after multiple in vitro subcultures. It was noted that treatment of *B henselae*-infected human beings with gentamicin in combination with amoxicillin or doxycycline is considered appropriate, and a combination of gentamicin with another antibiotic may be the treatment of choice for *Bartonella*-related endocarditis in people.[134-137] Investigators were unable to induce resistance in vitro to doxycycline or amoxicillin.[126-136]

Because of the uncertainty of antibiotic efficacy, and the concern that routine treatment of asymptomatic feline *Bartonella* infections may induce resistant strains, treatment can be recommended only for animals showing clinical signs of disease. Given the recent findings regarding induced resistance to antibiotics used to treat *Bartonella* infections, and data from experimental infections documenting efficacy of doxycycline treatment, the antibiotic of choice for treating ill cats may be doxycycline. Amoxicillin/clavulanic acid may have some efficacy.[95] Additional controlled studies are needed to assess antibiotic treatment protocols for *Bartonella* infections of pet animals.

Client education regarding the uncertainty of treatment efficacy is essential. The importance of flea control and other means of preventing transmission must be emphasized. In addition, the likelihood that cats may be readily reinfected with *Bartonella* following exposure to infected fleas, even if a *Bartonella* infection has been successfully treated, must be made clear to owners.

PREVENTION

Prevention of *Bartonella* infections is best accomplished by avoiding exposure to infected animals, fleas, and other arthropod vectors. Because *B henselae* and *B clarridgeiae* have been transmitted through inoculation of infected cat blood,[55] cats that are seropositive for *Bartonella* should not be used as blood donors. *B henselae* was reported to survive in stored human red blood cells for up to 35 days.[138] No vaccine is available to prevent *Bartonella* infection in cats.

PUBLIC HEALTH

Bartonella spp cause many clinical syndromes in human beings, some of which include CSD (typical and atypical forms, including encephalopathies in children and other neurologic abnormalities), bacillary angiomatosis, parenchymal bacillary peliosis, relapsing fever with bacteremia, endocarditis, optic neuritis, pulmonary, hepatic, or splenic granulomas, and osteomyelitis.[14,17,31,72,100,139–144] Immunocompetent individuals may have more localized infections, whereas infections that occur in immunocompromised individuals are more often systemic and can be fatal. Veterinarians, veterinary staff, groomers, and others with extensive companion animal contact are at a greater risk for *Bartonella* exposure than are members of the general public.[145,146] Veterinary staff should receive specific training regarding the zoonotic potential of *Bartonella* infections, and the potential modes of transmission.

Transmission of *B henselae* from cats to human beings probably occurs through contamination of cat scratches with flea excrement.[69] Transmission may occur through cat bites if cat blood or flea excrement contaminate the bite site or the cat's saliva. Ticks are considered possible vectors for transmission of some *Bartonella* infections, although their role in transmission of *Bartonella* infections remains undefined. Some persons with *Bartonella* infections have reported exposure to dogs and not cats, and others report no animal contact at all.[147–149]

The 2009 Guidelines for Preventing Opportunistic Infections Among HIV-infected Adults and Adolescents[150] recommend the following when acquiring a new cat: adopt a cat more than 1 year of age that is in good health, avoid rough play with cats, maintain flea control, wash any cat-associated wounds promptly, and do not allow cats to lick wounds or cuts. The Guidelines note no evidence that there is any benefit to cat owners from routine culture or serologic testing of healthy cats for *Bartonella*. However, because the negative predictive value of *B henselae* serology for feline bacteremia is good, serology may be an appropriate screening test for cats that immunocompromised persons are considering acquiring as pets. There is no evidence that declawing cats decreases the probability of transmission of *B henselae* from cats to human beings. Flea control is essential for interrupting transmission.

SUMMARY

The role of *Bartonella* species as feline pathogens is still an active area of investigation. Diagnosis and treatment of *Bartonella* infections remain challenging. It is recommended that the best practice for making a diagnosis of *Bartonella*-associated disease in cats is a combination of blood culture and/or PCR testing with serology and a careful evaluation for the presence of other potential causes for the clinical signs observed in a feline patient. Antibiotic treatment is recommended only if a cat is ill, and other potential causes for clinical signs are ruled out or treated. The most appropriate antibiotic treatment may be doxycycline, given its record of efficacy and the low likelihood that antibiotic resistance will develop.

Most *Bartonella* species infecting cats are zoonotic, with *B henselae* the most well recognized of these. *B henselae* bacteremia is common in domestic cats, and cats are an important vector for transmission to human beings. Transmission of *Bartonella* infections among cats primarily occurs via fleas, and fleas have a role in environmental contamination. Control of arthropod vectors, and avoiding interactions with pets that result in scratches or bites, are the most effective means currently available to prevent transmission among cats and between cats and human beings. Antibiotic treatment of healthy cats seropositive for *Bartonella* is not recommended, and may induce antibiotic-resistant strains.

As new information becomes available, our understanding of the complex pathogenesis of *Bartonella* infections continues to expand, and it is hoped that associations of feline *Bartonella* infection and clinical disease will become more clear.

REFERENCES

1. Brenner DJ, O'Connor SP, Winkler HH, et al. Proposals to unify the genera *Bartonella* and *Rochalimaea*, with descriptions of *Bartonella quintana* comb. nov., *Bartonella vinsonii* comb. nov., *Bartonella henselae* comb. nov., and *Bartonella elizabethae* comb. nov., and to remove the family *Bartonellaceae* from the order *Rickettsiales*. Int J Syst Bacteriol 1993;43:777–86.
2. Caceres-Rios H, Rodriguez-Tafur J, Bravo-Puccio F, et al. Verruga peruana: an infectious endemic angiomatosis. Crit Rev Oncog 1995;6(1):47–56.
3. Birtles RJ, Harrison TG, Saunders NA, et al. Proposals to unify the genera *Grahamella* and *Bartonella*, with descriptions of *Bartonella talpae* comb. nov., *Bartonella peromysci* comb. nov., and three new species, *Bartonella grahamii* sp. nov., *Bartonella taylorii* sp. nov., and *Bartonella doshiae* sp. nov. Int J Syst Bacteriol 1995;45(1):1–8.
4. Norman AF, Regnery R, Jameson P, et al. Differentiation of *Bartonella*-like isolates at the species level by PCR-restriction fragment length polymorphism in the citrate synthase gene. J Clin Microbiol 1995;33(7):1797–803.
5. Regnery RL, Anderson BE, Clarridge JE III, et al. Characterization of a novel *Rochalimaea* species, *R. henselae* sp. nov., isolated from blood of a febrile, human immunodeficiency virus-positive patient. J Clin Microbiol 1992;30(2): 265–74.
6. Weisburg WG, Woese CR, Dobson ME, et al. A common origin of rickettsiae and certain plant pathogens. Science 1985;230:556–8.
7. Johnson R, Ramos-Vara J, Vemulapalli R. Identification of *Bartonella henselae* in an aborted equine fetus. Vet Pathol 2009;46(2):277–81.
8. Jones SL, Maggi R, Shuler J, et al. Detection of *Bartonella henselae* in the blood of 2 adult horses. J Vet Intern Med 2008;22(2):495–8.
9. Maggi RG, Raverty SA, Lester SJ, et al. *Bartonella henselae* in captive and hunter-harvested beluga (*Delphinapterus leucas*). J Wildl Dis 2008;44(4):871–7.
10. Morick D, Osinga N, Gruys E, et al. Identification of a *Bartonella* species in the harbor seal (*Phoca vitulina*) and in sea lice (*Echinophtirius horridus*). Vector Borne Zoonotic Dis 2009;9(6):751–3.
11. Chomel BB, Kasten RW, Henn JB, et al. *Bartonella* infection in domestic cats and wild felids. Ann N Y Acad Sci 2006;1078:410–5.
12. Gillespie TN, Washabau RJ, Goldschmidt MH, et al. Detection of *Bartonella henselae* and *Bartonella clarridgeae* DNA in hepatic specimens from two dogs with hepatic disease. J Am Vet Med Assoc 2003;222(1):47–51.

13. Relman DA, Loutit JS, Schmidt TM, et al. The agent of bacillary angiomatosis: an approach to the identification of uncultured pathogens. N Engl J Med 1990; 323(23):1573–80.
14. Slater LN, Welch DF, Hensel D, et al. A newly recognized fastidious gram-negative pathogen as a cause of fever and bacteremia. N Engl J Med 1990;323: 1587–93.
15. Wong MT, Dolan MJ, Lattuada CP, et al. Neuroretinitis, aseptic meningitis, and lymphadenitis associated with *Bartonella (Rochalimaea) henselae* infection in immunocompetent patients and patients infected with human immunodeficiency virus type 1. Clin Infect Dis 1995;21(2):352–60.
16. De La Rosa GR, Barnett BJ, Ericsson CD, et al. Native valve endocarditis due to *Bartonella henselae* in a middle-aged human immunodeficiency virus-negative woman. J Clin Microbiol 2001;39(9):3417–9.
17. Fournier P-E, Lelievre H, Eykyn SJ, et al. Epidemiologic and clinical characteristics of *Bartonella quintana* and *Bartonella henselae* endocarditis: a study of 48 patients. Medicine 2001;80:245–51.
18. Gurfield AN, Boulouis H-J, Chomel BB, et al. Coinfection with *Bartonella clarridgeiae* and *Bartonella henselae* and with different *Bartonella henselae* strains in domestic cats. J Clin Microbiol 1997;35(8):2120–3.
19. Maruyama S, Nakamura Y, Kabeya H, et al. Prevalence of *Bartonella henselae*, *Bartonella clarridgeiae* and the 16S rRNA gene types of *Bartonella henselae* among pet cats in Japan. J Vet Med Sci 2000;62(3):273–9.
20. Kordick DL, Hilyard EJ, Hadfield TL, et al. Bartonella clarridgeiae, a newly recognized zoonotic pathogen causing inoculation papules, fever, and lymphadenopathy (cat scratch disease). J Clin Microbiol 1997;35(7):1813–8.
21. Lawson PA, Collins MD. Description of *Bartonella clarridgeiae* sp. nov. isolated from the cat of a patient with *Bartonella henselae* septicemia. Med Microbiol Lett 1996;5:64–73.
22. Chomel BB, MacDonald KA, Kasten RW, et al. Aortic valve endocarditis in a dog due to *Bartonella clarridgeiae*. J Clin Microbiol 2001;39(10):3548–54.
23. Droz S, Chi B, Horn E, et al. *Bartonella koehlerae* sp. nov., isolated from cats. J Clin Microbiol 1999;37(4):1117–22.
24. Avidor B, Graidy M, Efrat B, et al. *Bartonella koehlerae*, a new cat-associated agent of culture-negative human endocarditis. J Clin Microbiol 2004;42(8):3462–8.
25. Yamamoto K, Chomel BB, Kasten RW, et al. Experimental infection of domestic cats with *Bartonella koehlerae* and comparison of protein and DNA profiles with those of other *Bartonella* species infecting felines. J Clin Microbiol 2002;40(2): 466–74.
26. Ohad DG, Morick D, Avidor B, et al. Molecular detection of *Bartonella henselae* and *Bartonella* koehlerae from aortic valves of Boxer dogs with infective endocarditis. Vet Microbiol 2009;141:182–5.
27. Koehler JE. *Bartonella*-associated infections in HIV-infected patients. AIDS Clin Care 1995;7(12):97–102.
28. Koehler JE, Sanchez MA, Garrido CS, et al. Molecular epidemiology of *Bartonella* infections in patients with bacillary angiomatosis-peliosis. N Engl J Med 1997; 337(26):1876–83.
29. Breitschwerdt EB, Maggi RG, Sigmon B, et al. Isolation of *Bartonella quintana* from a woman and a cat following putative bite transmission. J Clin Microbiol 2007;45(1):270–2.
30. La VD, Tran-Hung L, Aboudharam G, et al. *Bartonella quintana* in domestic cat. Emerg Infect Dis 2005;11(8):1287–9.

31. Eremeeva ME, Gerns HL, Lydy SL, et al. Bacteremia, fever, and splenomegaly caused by a newly recognized *Bartonella* species. N Engl J Med 2007;356(23): 2381–7.

32. Henn JB, Chomel BB, Boulouis H-J, et al. *Bartonella rochalimae* in raccoons, coyotes, and red foxes. Emerg Infect Dis 2009;15(12):1984–7.

33. Henn JB, Gabriel MW, Kasten RW, et al. Infective endocarditis in a dog and the phylogenetic relationship of the associated "Bartonella rochalimae" strain with isolates from dogs, gray foxes, and a human. J Clin Microbiol 2009;47(3):787–90.

34. Chomel BB, Henn JB, Kasten RW, et al. Dogs are more permissive than cats or guinea pigs to experimental infection with a human isolate of *Bartonella rochalimae*. Vet Res 2009;40(4):27.

35. Regnery R, Martin M, Olson J. Naturally occurring "Rochalimaea henselae" infection in domestic cat. Lancet 1992;340:557–8.

36. Bermond D, Boulouis H-J, Heller R, et al. *Bartonella bovis* Bermond et al. sp. nov. and *Bartonella capreoli* sp. nov., isolated from European ruminants. Int J Syst Evol Microbiol 2002;52:383–90.

37. Koehler JE, Glaser CA, Tappero JW. *Rochalimaea henselae* infection: a new zoonosis with the domestic cat as reservoir. JAMA 1994;271:531–5.

38. Regnery R, Marano N, Jameson P, et al. A fourth *Bartonella* species, *Bartonella weissii*, species nova, isolated from domestic cats [abstract #4]. Proceedings of the 15th Sesquiannual Meeting American Society for Rickettsiology. Captiva Island (FL), April 30–May 3, 2000.

39. Jameson P, Greene C, Regnery R, et al. Prevalence of *Bartonella henselae* antibodies in pet cats throughout regions of North America. J Infect Dis 1995;172:1145–9.

40. Ueno H, Muramatsu Y, Chomel BB, et al. Seroepidemiological survey of *Bartonella (Rochalimaea) henselae* in domestic cats in Japan. Microbiol Immunol 1995;39:339–41.

41. Marston EL, Finlayson CJ, Regnery RL, et al. Prevalence of *Bartonella henselae* and *Bartonella clarridgeiae* in an urban Indonesian cat population. Clin Diagn Lab Immunol 1999;6(1):41–4.

42. Bergmans AM, DeJong CM, VanAmerongen G, et al. Prevalence of *Bartonella* species in domestic cats in the Netherlands. J Clin Microbiol 1997;35(9):2256–61.

43. Heller R, Artois M, Xemar V, et al. Prevalence of *Bartonella henselae* and *Bartonella clarridgeiae* in stray cats. J Clin Microbiol 1997;35(6):1327–31.

44. Nutter FB, Dubey JP, Levine JF, et al. Seroprevalence of antibodies against *Bartonella henselae* and *Toxoplasma gondii* and fecal shedding of *Cryptosporidium* spp, *Giardia* spp, and *Toxocara cati* in feral and pet domestic cats. J Am Vet Med Assoc 2004;225(11):1394–8.

45. Kordick DL, Papich MG, Breitschwerdt EB. Efficacy of enrofloxacin or doxycycline for treatment of *Bartonella henselae* or *Bartonella clarridgeiae* infection in cats. Antimicrob Agents Chemother 1997;41(11):2448–55.

46. Kordick DL, Wilson KH, Sexton DJ, et al. Prolonged *Bartonella* bacteremia in cats associated with cat-scratch disease patients. J Clin Microbiol 1995;33(12):3245–51.

47. Gurfield AN, Boulouis H-J, Chomel BB, et al. Epidemiology of Bartonella infection in domestic cats in France. Vet Microbiol 2001;80:185–98.

48. Chomel BB, Carlos ET, Kasten RW, et al. *Bartonella henselae* and *Bartonella clarridgeiae* infection in domestic cats from the Phillipines. Am J Trop Med Hyg 1999;60(4):593–7.

49. Rolain J-M, Franc M, Raoult D. First isolation and detection by immunofluorescence assay of Bartonella koehlerae in erythrocytes from a French cat. J Clin Microbiol 2003;41:4001–2.

50. Rotstein DS, Taylor SK, Bradley J, et al. Prevalence of *Bartonella henselae* antibody in Florida panthers. J Wildl Dis 2000;36(1):157–60.
51. Yamamoto K, Chomel BB, Lowenstine LJ, et al. *Bartonella henselae* antibody prevalence in free-ranging and captive wild felids from California. J Wildl Dis 1998;34(1):56–63.
52. Molia S, Chomel BB, Kasten RW, et al. Prevalence of *Bartonella* infection in wild African lions (*Panthera leo*) and cheetahs (*Acinonyx jubatus*). Vet Microbiol 2004;100:31–41.
53. Zeaiter Z, Fournier P-E, Raoult D. Genomic variation of *Bartonella henselae* strains detected in lymph nodes of patients with cat scratch disease. J Clin Microbiol 2002;40(3):1023–30.
54. Guptill L, Wu C-C, HogenEsch H, et al. Prevalence, risk factors, and genetic diversity of *Bartonella henselae* infections in pet cats in four regions of the United States. J Clin Microbiol 2004;42(2):652–9.
55. Kordick DL, Brown TT, Shin K, et al. Clinical and pathologic evaluation of chronic *Bartonella henselae* or *Bartonella clarridgeiae* infection in cats. J Clin Microbiol 1999;37(5):1536–47.
56. Berghoff J, Viezens J, Guptill L, et al. *Bartonella henselae* exists as a mosaic of different genetic variants in the infected host. Microbiology 2007;153(7): 2045–51.
57. Iredell J, Blanckenberg D, Arvand M, et al. Characterization of the natural population of *Bartonella henselae* by multilocus sequence typing. J Clin Microbiol 2003;41(11):5071–9.
58. Li W, Chomel BB, Maruyama S, et al. Multispacer typing to study the genotypic distribution of *Bartonella henselae* populations. J Clin Microbiol 2006;44(7): 2499–506.
59. Dillon B, Valenzuela J, Don R, et al. Limited diversity among human isolates of *Bartonella henselae*. J Clin Microbiol 2002;40(12):4691–9.
60. Maruyama S, Kasten RW, Boulouis H-J, et al. Genomic diversity of *Bartonella henselae* isolates from domestic cats from Japan, the USA and France by pulsed-field gel electrophoresis. Vet Microbiol 2000;79:337–49.
61. Kyme P, Dillon B, Iredell JR. Phase variation in *Bartonella henselae*. Microbiology 2003;149:621–9.
62. Iredell J, McHattan J, Kyme P, et al. Antigenic and genotypic relationships between *Bartonella henselae* strains. J Clin Microbiol 2002;40(11):4397–8.
63. Monteil M, Durand B, Bouchouicha R, et al. Development of discriminatory multiple-locus variable number tandem repeat analysis for *Bartonella henselae*. Microbiology 2007;153:1141–8.
64. Kabeya H, Maruyama S, Irei M, et al. Genomic variations among *Bartonella henselae* isolates derived from naturally infected cats. Vet Microbiol 2002;89:211–21.
65. Arvand M, Klose AJ, Schwartz-Porsche D, et al. Genetic variability and prevalence of *Bartonella henselae* in cats in Berlin, Germany, and analysis of its genetic relatedness to a strain from Berlin that is pathogenic for humans. J Clin Microbiol 2001;39(2):743–6.
66. Arvand M, Feil EJ, Giladi M, et al. Multi-locus sequence typing of *Bartonella henselae* isolates from three continents reveals hypervirulent and feline-associated clones. PLoS One 2007;2(12):e1346.
67. Chang C-C, Chomel BB, Kasten RW, et al. Molecular epidemiology of *Bartonella henselae* infection in human immunodeficiency virus-infected patients and their cat contacts, using pulsed-field gel electrophoresis and genotyping. J Infect Dis 2002;186:1733–9.

68. Chomel BB, Kasten RW, Floyd-Hawkins KA, et al. Experimental transmission of *Bartonella henselae* by the cat flea. J Clin Microbiol 1996;34(8):1952–6.

69. Foil L, Andress E, Freeland R, et al. Experimental infection of domestic cats with *Bartonella henselae* by inoculation of *Ctenocephalides felis* (Siphonaptera: Pulicidae) feces. J Med Entomol 1999;35(5):625–8.

70. Finkelstein JL, Brown TP, O'Reilly KL, et al. Studies on the growth of *Bartonella henselae* in the cat flea. J Med Entomol 2002;39(6):915–9.

71. Welch DF, Carroll KC, Hofmeister EK, et al. Isolation of a new subspecies, *Bartonella vinsonii* subsp. *arupensis*, from a cattle rancher: identity with isolates found in conjunction with *Borrelia burgdorferi* and *Babesia microti* among naturally infected mice. J Clin Microbiol 1999;37(8):2598–601.

72. Dietrich F, Schmidgen T, Maggi RG, et al. Prevalence of *Bartonella henselae* and *Borrelia burgdorferi* sensu lato DNA in *Ixodes ricinus* ticks in Europe. Appl Environ Microbiol 2010;76(5):1395–8.

73. Pappalardo BL, Correa MT, York CC, et al. Epidemiologic evaluation of the risk factors associated with exposure and seroreactivity to *Bartonella vinsonii* in dogs. Am J Vet Res 1997;58(5):467–71.

74. Chang CC, Chomel BB, Kasten RW, et al. Molecular evidence of *Bartonella* spp. in questing adult *Ixodes pacificus* ticks in California. J Clin Microbiol 2001;39(4):1221–6.

75. Chang C-C, Hayashidani H, Pusterla N, et al. Investigation of *Bartonella* infection in ixodid ticks from California. Comp Immunol Microbiol Infect Dis 2002;25:229–36.

76. Sanogo YO, Zeaiter Z, Caruso G, et al. *Bartonella henselae* in *Ixodes ricinus* ticks (Acari: Ixodida) removed from humans, Belluno Province, Italy. Emerg Infect Dis 2003;9(3):329–32.

77. Cotté V, Bonnet S, Le Rhun D, et al. Transmission of *Bartonella henselae* by *Ixodes ricinus*. Emerg Infect Dis 2008;14(7):1074–80.

78. Chung CY, Kasten RW, Paff SM, et al. *Bartonella* spp. DNA associated with biting flies from California. Emerg Infect Dis 2004;10(7):1311–3.

79. Telford SR 3rd, Wormser GP. Bartonella spp. transmission by ticks not established. Emerg Infect Dis 2010;16(3):679–84.

80. Bradbury C, Lappin MR. Evaluation of topical application of 10% imidacloprid-1% moxidectin to prevent *Bartonella henselae* transmission from cat fleas (*Ctenocephalides felis*) from cat fleas. J Am Vet Med Assoc 2010;236(8):869–73.

81. Guptill L, Slater L, Wu C-C, et al. Experimental infection of young specific pathogen-free cats with *Bartonella henselae*. J Infect Dis 1997;176:206–16.

82. Abbott RC, Chomel BB, Kasten RW, et al. Experimental and natural infection with *Bartonella henselae* in cats. Comp Immunol Microbiol Infect Dis 1997;20(1):41–57.

83. Kordick DL, Breitschwerdt EB. Relapsing bacteremia after blood transfusion of *Bartonella henselae* to cats. Am J Vet Res 1997;58(5):492–7.

84. Guptill L, Slater L, Wu C-C, et al. Evidence of reproductive failure and lack of perinatal transmission of *Bartonella henselae* in experimentally infected cats. Vet Immunol Immunopathol 1998;65:177–89.

85. Guptill L, Slater L, Wu C-C, et al. Immune response of neonatal specific pathogen-free cats to experimental infection with *Bartonella henselae*. Vet Immunol Immunopathol 1999;71:233–43.

86. Arvand M, Viezens J, Berghoff J. Prolonged *Bartonella henselae* bacteremia caused by reinfection in cats. Emerg Infect Dis 2008;14(1):152–4.

87. Kabeya H, Sase M, Yamashita M, et al. Predominant T helper 2 immune responses against *Bartonella henselae* in naturally infected cats. Microbiol Immunol 2006;50(3):171–8.

88. Kabeya H, Umehara T, Okanishi H, et al. Experimental infection of cats with *Bartonella henselae* resulted in rapid clearance associated with T helper 1 immune responses. Microbes Infect 2009;11(6–7):716–20.

89. Yamamoto K, Chomel BB, Kasten RW, et al. Homologous protection but lack of heterologous protection by various species and types of *Bartonella* in specific pathogen-free cats. Vet Immunol Immunopathol 1997;65:191–204.

90. Yamamoto K, Chomel BB, Kasten RW, et al. Infection and re-infection of domestic cats with various *Bartonella* species or types: *B. henselae* type I is protective against heterologous challenge with *B. henselae* type II. Vet Microbiol 2003;92:73–86.

91. Rolain JM, LaScola B, Davoust B, et al. Immunofluorescent detection of intraerythrocytic *Bartonella henselae* in naturally infected cats. J Clin Microbiol 2001; 39(8):2978–80.

92. Dehio C. *Bartonella* interactions with endothelial cells and erythrocytes. Trends Microbiol 2001;9(6):279–85.

93. Guptill L, Wu C-C, Glickman L, et al. Extracellular *Bartonella henselae* and artifactual intraerythrocytic pseudoinclusions in experimentally infected cats. Vet Microbiol 2000;76:283–90.

94. O'Reilly KL, Bauer RW, Freeland RL, et al. Acute clinical disease in cats following infection with a pathogenic strain of *Bartonella henselae* (LSU16). Infect Immun 1999;67(6):3066–72.

95. Greene CE, McDermott M, Jameson PH, et al. *Bartonella henselae* infection in cats: evaluation during primary infection, treatment, and rechallenge infection. J Clin Microbiol 1996;34(7):1682–5.

96. Mikolajczyk MG, O'Reilly KL. Clinical disease in kittens inoculated with a pathogenic strain of *Bartonella henselae*. Am J Vet Res 2000;61(4):375–9.

97. Lappin MR, Black JC. *Bartonella* spp infection as a possible cause of uveitis in a cat. J Am Vet Med Assoc 1999;214(8):1205–7.

98. Lappin MR, Kordick DL, Breitschwerdt EB. *Bartonella* spp. antibodies and DNA in aqueous humour of cats. J Feline Med Surg 2000;2:61–8.

99. Fontenelle JP, Powell CC, Hill AE, et al. Prevalence of serum antibodies against *Bartonella* species in the serum of cats with or without uveitis. J Feline Med Surg 2008;10:41–6.

100. Chomel BB, Kasten RW, Williams C, et al. *Bartonella* endocarditis: a pathology shared by animal reservoirs and patients. Ann N Y Acad Sci 2009;1166: 120–6.

101. Perez C, Hummel JB, Keene BW, et al. Successful treatment of Bartonella henselae endocarditis in a cat. J Fel Med Surg 2010;12(6):483–6.

102. Kirkpatrick CE, Moore FM, Patnaik AK, et al. Argyrophilic, intracellular bacteria in some cats with idiopathic peripheral lymphadenopathy. J Comp Pathol 1989; 101:341–9.

103. Bettenay SV, Lappin MR, Mueller RS. An immunohistochemical and polymerase chain reaction evaluation of feline plasmacytic pododermatitis. Vet Pathol 2007; 44:80–3.

104. Buchmann AU, Kempf VA, Kershaw O, et al. Peliosis hepatis in cats is not associated with *Bartonella henselae* infections. Vet Pathol 2010;47(1):163–6.

105. Ueno H, Hohdatsu T, Muramatsu Y, et al. Does coinfection of *Bartonella henselae* and FIV induce clinical disorders in cats? Microbiol Immunol 1996;40(9):617–20.

106. Glaus T, Hofmann-Lehmann R, Greene C, et al. Seroprevalence of *Bartonella henselae* infection and correlation with disease status in cats in Switzerland. J Clin Microbiol 1997;35(11):2883–5.

107. Dowers KL, Hawley JR, Brewer MM, et al. Association of *Bartonella* species, feline calicivirus, and feline herpesvirus 1 infection with gingivostomatitis in cats. J Feline Med Surg 2010;12(4):314–21.

108. Ishak AM, Radecki S, Lappin MR. Prevalence of *Mycoplasma haemofelis*, '*Candidatus* Mycoplasma haemominutum', *Bartonella* species, *Ehrlichia* species, and *Anaplasma phagocytophilum* DNA in the blood of cats with anemia. J Feline Med Surg 2007;9:1–7.

109. Pearce LK, Radecki SV, Brewer M, et al. Prevalence of *Bartonella henselae* antibodies in serum of cats with and without clinical signs of central nervous system disease. J Feline Med Surg 2006;8:315–20.

110. Quimby JM, Elston T, Hawley J, et al. Evaluation of the association of *Bartonella* species, feline herpesvirus 1, feline calicivirus, feline leukemia virus and feline immunodeficiency virus with chronic feline gingivostomatitis. J Feline Med Surg 2008;10:66–72.

111. Lappin MR, Breitschwerdt EB, Brewer M, et al. Prevalence of *Bartonella* species antibodies and *Bartonella* species DNA in the blood of cats with and without fever. J Feline Med Surg 2008;11(2):141–8.

112. Berryessa NA, Johnson LR, Kasten RW, et al. Microbial culture of blood samples and serologic testing for bartonellosis in cats with chronic rhinosinusitis. J Am Vet Med Assoc 2008;233(7):1084–9.

113. Bayliss D, Steiner JM, Sucholdolski JS, et al. Serum feline pancreatic lipase immunoreactivity concentration and seroprevalences of antibodies against *Toxoplasma gondii* and *Bartonella* species in client-owned cats. J Feline Med Surg 2009;11:663–7.

114. Chomel BB, Abbott RC, Kasten RW, et al. *Bartonella henselae* prevalence in domestic cats in California: risk factors and association between bacteremia and antibody titers. J Clin Microbiol 1995;33(9):2445–50.

115. Giladi M, Kletter Y, Avidor B, et al. Enzyme immunoassay for the diagnosis of cat-scratch disease defined by polymerase chain reaction. Clin Infect Dis 2001;33:1852–8.

116. Freeland RL, Scholl DT, Rohde KR, et al. Identification of *Bartonella*-specific immunodominant antigens recognized by the feline humoral immune system. Clin Diagn Lab Immunol 1999;6(4):558–66.

117. Birtles RJ, Laycock M, Kenny MJ, et al. Prevalence of *Bartonella* species causing bacteremia in domesticated and companion animals in the United Kingdom. Vet Rec 2002;151:225–9.

118. Maggi RG, Duncan AW, Breitschwerdt EB. Novel chemically modified liquid medium that will support the growth of seven *Bartonella* species. J Clin Microbiol 2005;43(6):2651–5.

119. Kamrani A, Parriera VR, Greenwood J, et al. The prevalence of *Bartonella*, hemoplasma, and *Rickettsia felis* infections in domestic cats and in cat fleas in Ontario. Can J Vet Res 2008;72:411–9.

120. Fenollar F, Raoult D. Molecular genetic methods for the diagnosis of fastidious microorganisms. APMIS 2004;112:785–807.

121. Lappin MR, Griffin B, Brunt J, et al. Prevalence of *Bartonella* species, haemoplasma species, *Ehrlichia* species, *Anaplasma phagocytophilum*, and *Neorickettsia risticii* DNA in the blood of cats and their fleas in the United States. J Feline Med Surg 2006;8:85–90.

122. Regnery RL, Rooney JA, Johnson AM, et al. Experimentally induced *Bartonella henselae* infections followed by challenge exposure and antimicrobial therapy in cats. Am J Vet Res 1996;57(12):1714–9.

123. Wiebe V. Fluoroquinolone-induced retinal degeneration in cats. J Am Vet Med Assoc 2002;221(11):1568–71.

124. Biswas S, Maggi RG, Papich MG, et al. Comparative activity of pradofloxacin, enrofloxacin and azithromycin against *Bartonella henselae* isolates derived from cats and a human. J Clin Microbiol 2010;48(2):617–8.

125. Angelakis E, Biswas S, Taylor C, et al. Heterogeneity of susceptibility to fluoro-quinolones in *Bartonella* isolates from Australia reveals a natural mutation in *gyrA*. J Antimicrob Chemother 2008;61:1252–5.

126. Biswas S, Raoult D, Rolain J-M. Molecular characterisation of resistance to rifampin in *Bartonella quintana*. Clin Microbiol Infect 2008;15(Suppl 2):100–1.

127. Bass JW, Freitas BC, Freitas AD, et al. Prospective randomized double blind placebo-controlled evaluation of azithromycin for treatment of cat-scratch disease. Pediatr Infect Dis J 1998;17(6):447–52.

128. Biswas S, Raoult D, Rolain J-M. Molecular characterization of resistance to macrolides in *Bartonella henselae*. Antimicrob Agents Chemother 2006; 50(9):3192–3.

129. Culic O, Erakovic V, Cepelak I, et al. Azithromycin modulates neutrophil function and circulating inflammatory mediators in healthy human subjects. Eur J Pharmacol 2002;450:277–89.

130. Labro MT. Interference of antibacterial agents with phagocyte functions: immunomodulation or "immuno-fairy tales"? Clin Microbiol Rev 2000;13(4):615–50.

131. Labro MT, Abdelghaffar H. Immunomodulation by macrolide antibiotics. J Chemother 2001;13(1):3–8.

132. Ortega E, Escobar A, Gaforia JJ, et al. Modification of phagocytosis and cytokine production in peritoneal and splenic cells by erythromycin A, azithromycin and josamycin. J Antimicrob Chemother 2004;53:367–70.

133. Meghari S, Rolain J-M, Grau GE, et al. Antiangiogenic effect of erythromycin: an in vitro model of *Bartonella quintana* infection. J Infect Dis 2006;193(1): 380–6.

134. Rolain JM, Brouqui P, Koehler JE, et al. Recommendations for treatment of human infections caused by *Bartonella* species. Antimicrob Agents Chemother 2004;48(6):1921–33.

135. Raoult D, Fournier PE, Vandenesch F, et al. Outcome and treatment of *Bartonella* endocarditis. Arch Intern Med 2003;163:226–30.

136. Biswas S, Raoult D, Rolain J-M. Molecular mechanism of gentamicin resistance in *Bartonella henselae*. Clin Microbiol Infect 2008;15(Suppl 2):98–9.

137. Habib G, Hoen G, Tornos P, et al. Guidelines on the prevention, diagnosis and treatment of infective endocarditis. Eur Heart J 2009;30:2369–413.

138. Magalhães RF, Urso Pitassi LH, Salvadego M, et al. *Bartonella henselae* survives after the storage period of red blood cell units: is it transmissible by transfusion? Transfus Med 2008;18(5):287–91.

139. Wheeler SW, Wolf SM, Steinberg EA. Cat-scratch encephalopathy. Neurology 1997;49:876–8.

140. Noah DL, Bresee JS, Gorensek MJ, et al. Cluster of five children with acute encephalopathy associated with cat-scratch disease in South Florida. Pediatr Infect Dis J 1995;14(10):866–9.

141. Margileth AM. Recent advances in diagnosis and treatment of cat scratch disease. Curr Infect Dis Rep 2000;2(2):141–6.

142. Roux V, Eykyn SJ, Wyllie S, et al. *Bartonella vinsonii* subsp. *berkhoffii* as an agent of afebrile blood culture-negative endocarditis in a human. J Clin Microbiol 2000;38(4):1698–700.

143. Spach DH, Koehler JE. *Bartonella*-associated infections. Infect Dis Clin North Am 1998;12(1):137–55.

144. Koehler JE, Sanchez MA, Tye S, et al. Prevalence of *Bartonella* infection among human immunodeficiency virus-infected patients with fever. Clin Infect Dis 2003; 37:559–66.

145. Noah DL, Kramer CM, Verbsky MP, et al. Survey of veterinary professionals and other veterinary conference attendees for antibodies to *Bartonella henselae* and *B. quintana*. J Am Vet Med Assoc 1997;210(3):342–4.

146. Kumasaka K, Arashima Y, Yanai M, et al. Survey of veterinary professionals for antibodies to *Bartonella henselae* in Japan. Rinsho Byori 2001;49:906–10.

147. Keret D, Giladi M, Kletter Y, et al. Cat-scratch osteomyelitis from a dog scratch. J Bone Joint Surg Br 1998;80:766–7.

148. Tsukahara M, Tsuneoka H, Iino H, et al. *Bartonella henselae* infection from a dog. Lancet 1998;352:1682.

149. Hadfield TL, Warren R, Kass M, et al. Endocarditis caused by *Rochalimaea henselae*. Hum Pathol 1993;24(10):1140–1.

150. Kaplan AJ, Benson C, Holmes KK, et al. Guidelines for prevention and treatment of opportunistic infections in HIV-infected adults and adolescents. MMWR Recomm Rep 2009;58(RR04):1–198.

Canine Leptospirosis

Richard E. Goldstein, DVM

KEYWORDS

• Leptospira • Spirochete • Canine • Infectious disease
• Zoonosis

ETIOLOGY

Leptospirosis is a disease of humans and animals caused by infection with the motile spirochetal bacterium of the genus, *Leptospira*.[1] Leptospirosis as a zoonotic disease worldwide cannot be overstated, because it causes human disease and deaths in much of the world, but mostly in areas of Asia and South America. The bacteria are highly motile, thin, flexible, and filamentous, made up of fine spirals with hook-shaped ends. Motility is gained by writhing and flexing movements while rotating along the long axis.[1] The bacterium is an obligate aerobic spirochete that share features of both gram-negative and gram-positive bacteria.

Many classification methods have been used to divide up the pathogenic leptospires into more workable groups. An antigenic classification schemed used in the past divided them into distinct serogroups based on surface antigens, each containing one or more serovar. Newer classification schemes are based on genetic methodologies. Today, most of the commonly diagnosed canine pathogenic serovars are still classified (as before) as belonging to the *Leptospira interrogans* species, although the common canine serovar grippotyphosa is typically classified as belonging to the *L kirschneri* species.[1]

Approximately 250 different serovars have been identified in the *Leptospira* complex.[2] Many of the isolates are of unknown clinical importance in any species. Six to eight serovars are thought pathogenic in the dog.[3–5] Each serovar has a primary or definitive host that maintains the organism and contributes to its dissemination in the environment. Although all mammals may be susceptible to infection, clinical signs are expected to be most severe with non–host-adapted serovars, whereas the definitive host is typically infected at a young age and is thought to most commonly exhibit minimal clinical disease.[6]

Canine leptospirosis was first described in 1899. Before 1960, *L interrogans* serovars icterohaemorrhagiae and canicola were believed responsible for most clinical cases of canine leptospirosis. The disease then, mainly described as acute or subacute hepatic and renal failure, was often thought characterized by acute hemorrhagic diathesis,

Department of Clinical Sciences, College of Veterinary Medicine, Cornell University, Ithaca, NY 14853, USA
E-mail address: Rg225@cornell.edu

Vet Clin Small Anim 40 (2010) 1091–1101
doi:10.1016/j.cvsm.2010.07.008
0195-5616/10/$ – see front matter © 2010 Published by Elsevier Inc.

icterus, or uremia.[7] Because these serovars were considered the most common in dogs, they are also the ones found in the long-existing bivalent vaccines. After these vaccines came into widespread use, the incidence of classic leptospirosis in dogs, from these two serovars, seems to have decreased,[8] although a cause and effect between the widespread use of the vaccine and the reduction of infection with these serovars has not been proved. In the past 20 years, several reports of increased incidence of the disease have been published with only a few cases of those classic serovars in North America in dogs (**Table 1**). The most common serovars today in the United States in reports are thought to be *L kirschneri* serovar grippotyphosa, *L interrogans* serovar pomona, and *L interrogans* serovar *bratislava*.[6,7,9] The recent increase in the diagnosis of the disease seems real, not just an effect of increased testing.[9] Beginning in 2000, new vaccines have appeared on the market that include *Leptospira* serovars grippotyphosa and pomona. It is likely too soon to assess a potential serovar shift, if there is one, after the use of the newer vaccines. In recent years, increasing incidence of dogs testing serologically positive to *L kirschneri* serovar autumnalis has also been documented as many commercial laboratories have added this serovar to their testing panel.[9,10] Little is known about this serovar in the dog in terms of experimental infection, and it may emerge as an important cause of renal and nonrenal leptospirosis in the future, but it also seems a common serologic result even in vaccinated research dogs and in other dogs that have not been exposed to this serovar.[11,12] Recent reviews assessing suspected serovar incidence in confirmed cases of leptospirosis in different regions of North America (see **Table 1**). Results of many reviews need to be examined carefully, however, because they are usually based on serosurveys typically using the microscopic agglutination test (MAT), which is likely a poor predictor of the true infecting serovar. Other serovars have been documented in different parts of the world. Serogroup Australis has also been incriminated in an outbreak in Canada and has been documented as the cause of chronic hepatitis in dogs in France and leptospirosis in Italy. In Germany, the predominant serovars seem to be grippotyphosa, saxkoebing, icterohaemorrhagiea, canicola, and bratislava; a recent survey in Italy identified serovars bratislava and grippotyphosa.[7,8,13–18]

EPIDEMIOLOGY

There are two types of mammalian hosts when it comes to *Leptospira* infections. Each serovar is adapted to one or more mammals as a primary, also called the definitive or

---

Table 1
Recent reviews documenting the most common serovars in dogs with leptospirosis from different areas of North America

First Author (Region)	Journal	Year	No. of Cases	Predominant Serovars
Goldstein (New York)	JVIM	2006	55	Grippotyphosa Pomona
Ward (Indiana)	JAVMA	2004	90	Grippotyphosa
Prescott (Ontario)	Can Vet J	2002	31	Autumnalis Bratislava
Adin (California)	JAVMA	2000	36	Pomona Bratislava
Ribotta (Quebec)	Can Vet J	2000	19	Prippotyphosa Pomona

Data from Goldstein RE. Leptospirosis—epidemiology, pathogenesis, and zoonotic impact on veterinary practices. Insights Vet Med 2007;5(2):2.

reservoir, host. Adapted resevoir hosts are thought to harbor persistent infection, often without severe signs of disease and can shed organisms in their urine for months to years after infection. The bacteria are maintained in the renal tubules of reservoir hosts and excreted in the urine. The other type of mammalian host is the incidental host that becomes infected with a specific serovar that is not adapted to living chronically in this species of mammal. Incidental hosts tend to develop clinical disease and either clears the organisms or die; rarely do they develop a chronic carrier state.

The dog serves as the reservoir host only for the pathogenic *L interrogans* serovar canicola. The reservoir hosts for the other serovars include common rodents, skunks, raccoons, farm animals, and deer, which can carry and excrete the bacteria in their urine for extended periods.[3] The incidence of the canine chronic carrier state for *Leptospira* organisms is unknown. If this state exists, it is likely to specifically exist for dogs infected with *L interrogans* serovar canicola. It is less likely, and even less clear, whether or not such a carrier state exists in dogs infected with other serovars that have not adapted for persistence in the dog and are more commonly seen at least in the ill canine population today.

Leptospires can be transmitted directly between hosts in close contact through urine, venereal routes, placental transfer, bites, or ingestion of infected tissues as the organism penetrates mucosa or broken skin. Shedding by infected animals occurs, usually via urine. The exact duration of shedding and potential spread to other dogs or humans is uncertain and may depend on the serovar. Indirect transmission, which probably happens more frequently, occurs through exposure of susceptible animals or humans to a contaminated environment, where the organisms persist after exposure from the urine of an infected host. Water contact is the most common means of spread, and habitats with stagnant or slow-moving warm water favor organism survival. Even in rapid moving water, however, it seems that the organism survives in high concentration in the shallow areas or adheres to rocks and other debris.

The invasion of the *Leptospira* organisms into the host is via skin wounds or through intact mucous membranes. The organism survives only transiently in undiluted acidic urine (pH 5.0 to 5.5) as neutral to basic pH is favorable for its survival. Dilute or non-concentrated urine provides a suitable habitat. Freezing markedly decreases survival of the organism outside the host, likely contributing to a seasonal pattern of infection in colder climates. Ambient temperatures between 0°C and 25°C favor survival of the organism, Therefore, rainfall, temperature, and pH requirements may explain the apparent increased incidence of canine leptospirosis in late summer and early fall, In the southern, semitropical belt of the United States, and in similar climatic regions worldwide. Seasonality in many parts of the country is associated with rainfall.[6,19–21] Reports exist of disease outbreaks occurring during or immediately after periods of flooding. In a large recent human outbreak in triatheletes in Illinois, people became infected after swimming in a lake a short time after strong rains and flooding occurred, which likely washed bacteria into the shallow areas of the lake creating puddles on the shore that had been contaminated from raccoon urine.[22]

After penetration in a susceptible host, leptospires begin to multiply as early as 1 day after entering the blood vascular space.[23] This initiates a leptospiremic phase, which lasts a few days involving rapid replication of the bacteria and endothelial damage. After this phase, invasion of a variety of end organs, including the kidneys, liver, spleen, central nervous system (CNS), eyes, and genital tract can occur. Leptospires damage organs by replicating and inducing cytokine production and inflammatory cell invasion. The initial replication mainly damages the endothelial cells and only later the kidneys and liver. The extent of damage to internal organs varies seems to depend on the virulence of the organism, including serovar and strain, the inoculum, and host susceptibility.[24]

Recovery from infection seems to depend on the production of specific antibodies. As serum antibodies increase, the organism is thought to be cleared. Based on experimental studies, renal colonization occurs in most infected dogs that do not have adequate protection from prior exposure or vaccination. Data are lacking regarding the incidence of chronic renal colonization in naturally infected dogs.

PATHOGENESIS

The sequence of events after infection seems amazingly variable and likely depends on

- Virulence, serovar, and perhaps even strain in addition to numbers of bacteria infecting the host. The author and colleagues have recently shown that suspected L interrogans serovar pomona infections induced significantly more severe kidney disease and had a worse outcome than infection suspected to be from other serovars in a study of naturally occurring leptospirosis in dogs in New York State.[7]
- Immune response. Previous exposure (naturally occurring or vaccinal) to the same serovar is likely to provide some degree of immunity although the duration of immunity after natural infection and the degree of cross protection between serovars are unknown in dogs. Immunity, however, is not predicted by MAT titers and seems to last at least 1 year after vaccination. A recent study comparing different commercially available vaccines showed only a mild serologic response to a series of two vaccinations but good immunity when challenged 1 year after the second vaccine.[25]

After the leptospiremic phase, the following organs are typically targeted by the bacteria:

- The kidneys: renal colonization occurs in most experimentally infected dogs.[25] Organisms persist and multiply in the tubular aspect of the renal tubular epithelial cells causing cytokine release, inflammatory cell recruitment, and acute nephritis. It is unclear how often this leads to the development of a chronic carrier state with urinary shedding. The likelihood of this occurring is thought significantly higher when the infecting serovar is canicola, because it is adapted to the dog as the primary host. Interstitial nephritis may be a chronic manifestation of acute disease in dogs
- The liver: centrilobular necrosis and subcellular damage, bile canaliculi, and duct occlusion are thought to occur and may cause icterus. This was thought a common occurrence in serovar icterohaemorrhagiae and may not be as common today[7]
- Endothelium: tissue edema and disseminated intravascular coagulation may occur within the first few days of infection as a result an acute endothelial injury.[26]
- Additional body systems may also be damaged during the acute phase of infection. A benign meningitis is produced when leptospires invade the CNS. The incidence in dogs of CNS involvement is unknown; however, it is well documented in humans. Uveitis may occur in naturally occurring and experimentally induced canine leptospirosis in addition to abortion and infertility resulting from transplacental transmission of leptospires.[26] Pulmonary manifestations can be severe in canine leptospirosis. Clinically, these dogs experience labored respiration and coughing. Lung changes in dogs with leptospirosis are associated with pulmonary hemorrhage, most likely due to endothelial damage and vasculitis.[24] Secondary immune-mediated disease (polyarthritis, hemolytic anemia, and so forth) has been suspected to occur but the true incidence of canine cases is unknown.[26]

DIAGNOSIS

Achieving as definitive a diagnosis as possible should be of special importance to veterinary practitioners because of the zoonotic potential of the disease and the possibility of the dog serving as a reservoir for other dogs and humans. Unfortunately, achieving a definitive diagnosis is often difficult with the tools in use today. The first difficulty faced is that the clinical signs associated with this disease are often vague and are typically nonspecific. The clinicopathologic data are often more of a function of the end-organ damage and nonspecific as well. Subtle abnormalities and combinations of abnormal clinicopathologic data are often the key for a high index of suspicion necessary in these cases. Specific leptospirosis testing in practice today is typically still limited to serology although PCR testing may become a more common modality in the future, especially for acute cases. The MAT serologic test commonly used today lacks both sensitivity (negative results early in the disease process) and specificity (reacts positively with vaccinal antibodies) when a single test is performed. Thus, a high index of suspicion is required and veterinarians most often have to submit repeated samples to obtain a definitive diagnosis.

SIGNALMENT AND HISTORY

Identifying dogs more likely to become infected with *Leptospira* organisms is important to narrow down the need for specific and sometimes expensive and repetitive testing. A profile of the kind of dog more likely to be infected is also beneficial when deciding which dogs should be vaccinated against the disease. There are likely large geographic differences in these considerations and so the region and season should be taken into account, although large amounts of epidemiologic data by region are lacking for most areas.[27] Roaming dogs and dogs exposed to standing water possibly contaminated by wildlife urine are more likely to be exposed. Some studies suggest male dogs are more likely to develop the disease possibly for that reason.[21,26] Anecdotally, however, it seems that even small dogs in some urban environments contract the disease, forcing veterinary practitioners to be aware of possible regional differences, to maintain a wide index of suspicion, and to think broadly when dogs present with appropriate clinical signs and when making vaccine decisions.

CLINICAL SIGNS

Clinical signs of dogs with leptospirosis can vary from subclinical or minimal clinical disease or mild fever to severe kidney, liver, and pulmonary disease. The literature is biased by the testing that was performed in each study, meaning that if only test azotemic dogs are tested, then all dogs diagnosed will be azotemic. It seems, however, that subtle to severe signs of kidney and liver damage as well as coagulation defects predominate. It is unknown what percentage of naïve naturally infected dogs show obvious clinical signs, because subclinical disease is common in experimental infections. Peracute leptospiral infections have been produced experimentally[28] and were characterized by massive leptospiremia, causing shock and often death. It is unknown how common this disease course is in naturally occurring cases. In a recent study of naturally occurring cases in New York State, the most common clinical signs included lethargy, vomiting, anorexia, and polydipsia. Abdominal pain, polyuria, and polydipsia were often striking in their magnitude. Overt icterus and fever on initial presentation were uncommon clinical signs and should not be relied on to determine which dogs should be tested for the disease.[7]

CLINICOPATHOLOGIC DATA

Unfortunately there are few or no single clinicopathologic changes on a chemistry panel, complete blood count (CBC), or urine analysis that are pathognomonic for leptospirosis. Practitioners must take multiple, often subtle, abnormalities into account to try and build a case for the diagnosis of this disease in dogs. The most common abnormalities found in the chemistry panel of confirmed cases include azotemia, increased serum liver enzyme activity, electrolyte disturbances, and mild increases in serum bilirubin concentrations. Coagulation parameters may be altered in severely affected animals. The CBC abnormalities often include a mild to moderate leukocytosis and thrombocytopenia. Thus, a combination of these CBC abnormalities and azotemia or increased liver enzymes should be suggestive of leptospirosis. Signs of acute tubular injury, such as mild proteinuria and glucosuria, are often found on the urine analysis.[7,26]

IMAGING

As in many types of infectious disease, imaging modalities of radiographs and ultrasound are helpful in ruling out additional causes of the clinical disease but are less helpful in confirming a diagnosis of leptospirosis. Characteristic changes have been described in the lungs on thoracic radiographs[29,30] and in the kidneys on abdominal ultrasound[31] in dogs with leptospirosis. Both of these studies were retrospective uncontrolled case series and it is unclear how often or how specific these findings are in dogs with this disease.

Thus, the decision to submit specific tests to attempt to confirm the diagnosis of leptospirosis is made based on the clinical picture that combines data from signalment, history, physical examination, and a broad minimal database. **Fig. 1** represents a possible approach for diagnosing canine leptospirosis.

SPECIFIC TESTING

The most commonly used test today in veterinary practice in North America is the MAT.[26] This test is performed by mixing serial dilutions of the canine sera with cultured *Leptospira* organisms of different serovars representing different serogroups. The titer against a specific serogroup is defined as the highest dilution of the sera that caused 50% or more agglutination of the organisms representing that serogroup. There are many inherent problems with the performance of this test. One is the possibility of subclinical infections and the persistence of antibodies, such that a positive test does not confirm disease. Perhaps more importantly, specifically for the diagnosis of leptospirosis, the MAT test does not differentiate between antibodies produced as a result of true exposure to the organism and antibodies produced after vaccination. An additional serious limitation to the diagnosis of leptospirosis with a single MAT titer is that in many cases this titer is negative at the time of initial presentation, falsely ruling out the disease if a single early titer is relied on. Negative initial antibody tests can be explained by the 7- to 9-day period required before MAT antibodies are detected. MAT titers become positive after approximately I week, peak at 3 to 4 weeks, and remain positive for months after both natural infection and vaccination.[26] It has been assumed that a high MAT titer ($\geq$800) to a nonvaccinal serovar and a negative or low ($\leq$400) titers against vaccinal serovars, accompanied by clinical signs of leptospirosis, is typically considered highly suggestive of active infection.[26] Although, in two studies where naïve puppies were given two different quadrivalent leptospiral vaccines, the MAT titers were often high or even the highest to the nonvaccinal serovar

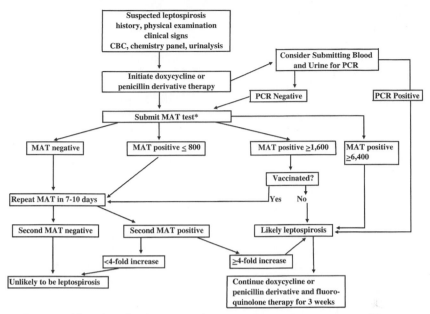

Fig. 1. Suggested flowchart for the current diagnosis of canine leptospirosis using the MAT. (*) Recommended serovars for testing in North America include grippotyphosa, pomona, bratislava, canicola, icterohemorrhagiae, and autumnalis. (*From* Goldstein RE. Leptospirosis in veterinary internal medicine expert consult. In: Ettinger SJ, Feldman EC, editors. Textbook of veterinary internal medicine expert consult. 7th edition. Saunders; 2010: p. 866 (Fig. 198–1); with permission.)

autumnalis[30] (Midence and colleagues, ACVIM 2010[12]). Therefore, a single reliable titer may only be when it is greater than 1:3200 for a vaccinal serovar and greater than 1:1600 for a nonvaccinal serovar.[26] Another potential use of MAT titers is deciphering the likely infecting serogroup based on the serovar that gives the highest titer. This task is made difficult because of the large degree of cross-reactivity among serogroups so that the highest titers to a specific serogroup may not definitely identify the causative serovar. In a human study where urine cultures and MAT results were compared, the MAT accurately predicted serovar in only 46% of the cases.[32] Another cofounding factor in the interpretation of the MAT test is the large degree of interlaboratory variation.[26] Fortunately for veterinary practitioners, however, knowing the infecting serovar is not crucial information necessary for an appropriate diagnosis or treatment. It seems that all common serovars today in the dog population cause a clinically similar disease that is treated in an identical fashion regardless of the serovar.[7,17] These data are important, however, from an epidemiologic and vaccine development standpoint.

Given these limitations of a single MAT titer, perhaps the most reliable way to use this test is to routinely perform a convalescent titer. A 4-fold change in a MAT convalescent tier when compared with baseline titers is consistent with active infection. Because antibody test results are often negative in the first week of illness, especially in young dogs (<6 months of age), a second serum sample should be obtained within I to 2 weeks. Therefore, to confirm current infection versus previous infection or vaccination, a change in titer should be demonstrated. Antimicrobial therapy early in the course of the disease may decrease the magnitude of the titer rise; therefore, the second sample should be obtained at 1 to 2 weeks after the first and not the typical 3-week convalescent window.

Direct isolation or identification of organisms is often the ideal mode of diagnosis in infectious disease. Direct culture of the organism from blood or urine is the gold standard. Unfortunately this is almost never performed in clinical veterinary medicine. The organism itself is hard to culture, requiring immediate placement in a special medium before any antibiotic therapy. Thus cultures cannot be performed on previously shipped urine at a referral laboratory. Cultures are also expensive and expose laboratory workers to possible exposure to the organism. Despite this, cultures should be encouraged in veterinary medicine because the data derived from culture confirmed cases are superior to those derived from serologically confirmed cases.

Direct visualization of the *Leptospira* organisms is possible in some cases. Darkfield microscopy has been used in the past in veterinary medicine for the diagnosis of leptospirosis in large and small animals. Unfortunately, this method lacks sensitivity and specificity and is not recommended today.[33] Identification of the organism in paraffin-embedded tissue can sometimes be accomplished using Giemsa or modified Steiner (silver) stain, immunofluorescence, or immunohistochemistry. Because leptospirosis cases are rarely biopsied antemortem, these techniques on tissue are usually only made post mortem. Their use in body fluids, however, such as urine, when large amounts or organisms are present is possible as well.[34] Polymerase chain reaction (PCR) is becoming a more common modality in the diagnosis of infectious diseases. Real-time PCR is the most sensitive and is currently commercially available in the United States. A combination of testing, both blood and urine, before antibiotic therapy is ideal because blood samples tend to be positive early in infection and then later the urine becomes positive.[35] In two studies comparing PCR, culture, and antibody testing in healthy and diseased animals, PCR was significantly more sensitive than the other methods in identifying shedders and diagnosing the disease.[36,37] Because of all the limitations of culturing, PCR may become the best approach for direct detection of the organism in the future, especially when testing for subclinical infection or chronic shedding. Recent advances in PCR techniques have allowed not only diagnosis of leptospirosis but also perhaps identification of specific *Leptospira* serovars.[38] The use of real-time PCR is possible even in recently vaccinated dogs. In a recent study, two real-time PCR were not influenced by vaccinal DNA in these dogs.[12] More data are required regarding the sensitivity and specificity of PCR in large numbers of naturally occurring cases before its true value its known. The current recommendation is to submit blood and urine before antibiotic therapy. **Fig. 1** shows a possible diagnostic algorithm combining PCR and serologic diagnostics.

TREATMENT

Treatment of leptospirosis involves supportive care, treating the renal or hepatic manifestations of the disease, and the use of antimicrobials. Antimicrobial therapy should be started as soon as the disease is suspected and samples have been drawn (if PCR is submitted). This is essential to eliminate bacteremia and the potential for live organisms in the urine that pose a zoonotic risk to humans. This should be started before confirmation of the diagnosis. A study in humans revealed that if antibiotics were delayed by 7 days after presentation, there was no longer an advantage to their administration.[39] The eventual goal of therapy is also to clear the organisms from tissue in addition to the blood and urine. The first goal of terminating bacteremia and sterilizing the urine can be achieved with doxycycline or a penicillin derivative. Doxycycline seems the drug of choice for the clearing of the organism from tissue. Therefore, when the disease is suspected, if oral drugs can be administered, then doxycycline (5 mg/kg every 12 hours) or amoxicillin (22 mg/kg every 12 hours) can be used at that time. Ampicillin (22 mg/kg intravenously every 8 hours) or amoxicillin, if available for intravenous use (22 mg/kg every 12 hours), is preferred for dogs that cannot be given oral drugs initially. Shedding should be terminated within 24 hours of initiating antibiotics, greatly reducing the risk to humans and other dogs. Doxycycline (5 mg/kg orally every 12 hours for 3 weeks) is the drug of choice for clearing the organism from tissue or eliminating the carrier state. Doxycycline treatment should start as soon as oral therapy is possible if not used intravenously. Therefore, in a suspected case of leptospirosis, the common protocols include doxycycline alone for all animals that can tolerate oral therapy or a penicillin derivative that is switched to doxycycline after the diagnosis has been confirmed and the dog can tolerate oral medications.

Aggressive fluid therapy concurrent to the use of antibiotics is crucial to prevent and treat acute kidney damage. The extent of renal damage after treatment may play a key role in determining the long-term prognosis for affected dogs. Hemodialysis has been beneficial in dogs that develop anuria or oliguria or are refractive to fluid therapy.[6] Some dogs have an apparent clinical recovery after treatment, whereas others develop persistent azotemia with an overall survival rate approaching 80% in most studies.[6,7]

PREVENTION

Prevention ideally should start by limiting contact of pet dogs with wild animal reservoirs of the disease as well as sources of contaminated water. This is, of course, easier said than done, given the close contact of pets to wild animals, including rodents, even in urban areas. Thus vaccination is crucial to prevent the disease in at-risk dogs. All available vaccines are culture based and contained whole units or subunits of inactivated bacterins of serovars icterohaemorrhagiae and canicola. It is assumed, however, that these vaccines are not cross-protective against the serovars responsible for most of the current infections in dogs. To date, two bacterin-based vaccines that also contain serovars grippotyphosa and pomona as quadrivalent products are now on the market in the United States. These vaccines are recommended used annually after a two-injection initial series in a puppy or previously unvaccinated dog. Good protection has been shown to persist for 1 year despite very low MAT antibody titers at the time of challenge for other bacterin type of vaccines containing serovars icterohaemorrhagiae and canicola[25]; recently, similar results have been presented regarding serovar grippotyphosa.[40] Anecdotally, leptospiral vaccines have been thought to have a high incidence of allergenic reactions, especially in certain breeds, such as dachshunds and pugs. In a recent study, however, a quadrivalent leptospiral vaccine was not more reactive than other bacterin-based vaccines, including the vaccine used to prevent Lyme disease.[41]

SUMMARY

Leptospirosis is a common zoonotic disease with a worldwide distribution. Dogs become infected by exposure to contaminated urine from shedding wild animals. The bacteria penetrate mucus membranes cause endothelial damage in organs, such as the liver and kidneys. The clinical signs and clinicopathologic data are nonspecific and a high index of suspicion is needed by practitioners. Testing today is highly based on serology (MAT) and perhaps PCR. Treatment of leptospirosis involves supportive care and antibiotics, and prevention includes environmental steps and annual vaccination of dogs at risk.

REFERENCES

1. Bharti AR, Nally JE, Ricaldi JN, et al. Leptospirosis: a zoonotic disease of global importance. Lancet Infect Dis 2003;3(12):757–71.
2. Levett PN. Leptospirosis. Clin Microbiol Rev 2001;14:296–326.
3. Baldwin CJ, Atkins CE. Leptospirosis in dogs. Compendium on Continuing Education for the Practicing Veterinarian 1987;9:499–507.
4. Friedland JS, Warrell DA. The Jarisch-Herxheimer reaction in leptospirosis: possible pathogenesis and review. Rev Infect Dis 1991;13:207–10.
5. Adin CA, Cowgill LD. Treatment and outcome of dogs with leptospirosis: 36 cases (1990–1998). J Am Vet Med Assoc 2000;216:371–5.
6. Goldstein RE, Lin RC, Langston CE, et al. Influence of infecting serogroup on clinical features of leptospirosis in dogs. J Vet Intern Med 2006;20(3):489–94.
7. Brown CA, Roberts AW, Miller MA, et al. *Leptospira interrogans* serovar grippotyphosa infection in dogs. J Am Vet Med Assoc 1996;209:1265–7.
8. Rentko VT, Clark N, Ross LA, et al. Canine leptospirosis: a retrospective study of 17 cases. J Vet Intern Med 1992;6:235–44.
9. Moore GE, Guptill LF, Glickman NW, et al. Canine leptospirosis, United States, 2002-2004. Emerg Infect Dis 2006;12(3):501–3.
10. Prescott JF, McEwen B, Taylor J, et al. Resurgence of leptospirosis in dogs in Ontario: recent findings. Can Vet J 2002;43:955–61.
11. Barr SC, McDonough PL, Scipioni-Ball RL, et al. Serologic responses of dogs given a commercial vaccine against *Leptospira interrogans* serovar pomona and *Leptospira kirschneri* serovar grippotyphosa. Am J Vet Res 2005;66(10): 1780–4.
12. Midence JN, Chandler AM, Goldstein RE. Assessing the effect of recent Leptospira vaccination on whole blood real time PCR testing in dogs [abstract]. In: Forum of the American College of Veterinary Internal Medicine, 2010.
13. Nielsen JN, Cochran GK, Cassells JA, et al. *Leptospira interrogans* serovar bratislava infection in two dogs. J Am Vet Med Assoc 1991;199:351–2.
14. Scanziani E, Crippa L, Giusti AM, et al. *Leptospira interrogans* serovar sejroe infection in a group of laboratory dogs. Lab Anim 1995;29:300–6.
15. Harkin KR, Gartrell CL. Canine leptospirosis in New Jersey and Michigan: 17 cases (1990–1995). J Am Anim Hosp Assoc 1996;32:495–501.
16. Birnbaum N, Barr SC, Center SA, et al. Naturally acquired leptospirosis in 36 dogs: serological and clinicopathological features. J Small Anim Pract 1998;39:231–6.
17. Geisen V, Stengel C, Brem S, et al. Canine leptospirosis infections—clinical signs and outcome with different suspected *Leptospira* serogroups (42 cases). J Small Anim Pract 2007;48(6):324–8.
18. Scanziani E, Origgi F, Giusti AM, et al. Serological survey of leptospiral infection in kennelled dogs in Italy. J Small Anim Pract 2002;43:154–7.
19. Ward MP. Seasonality of canine leptospirosis in the United States and Canada and its association with rainfall. Prev Vet Med 2002;56:203–13.
20. Ward MP. Clustering of reported cases of leptospirosis among dogs in the United States and Canada. Prev Vet Med 2002;56:215–26.
21. Ward MP, Glickman LT, Guptill LE. Prevalence of and risk factors for leptospirosis among dogs in the United States and Canada: 677 cases (1970–1998). J Am Vet Med Assoc 2002;220:53–8.
22. Morgan J, Bornstein SL, Karpati AM, et al. Outbreak of leptospirosis among triathlon participants and community residents in Springfield, Illinois, 1998. Clin Infect Dis 2002;34(12):1593–9.

23. Saravanan R, Rajendran P, Garajan SP. Clinical, bacteriologic, and histopathologic studies on induced leptospirosis in stray dog pups. Indian J Pathol Microbiol 1999;42:463–9.
24. Midwinter A, Vinh T, Faine S, et al. Characterization of an antigenic oligosaccharide from *Leptospira interrogans* serovar pomona and its role in immunity. Infect Immun 1994;62:5477–82.
25. Klaasen HL, Molkenboer MJ, Vrijenhoek MP, et al. Duration of immunity in dogs vaccinated against leptospirosis with a bivalent inactivated vaccine. Vet Microbiol 2003;95(1-2):121–32.
26. Greene EC, Sykes JE, Brown CA, et al. Leptospirosis. In: Greene CD, editor. Infectious diseases of the dog and the cat. 3rd edition. St Louis (MO): Saunders-Elsevier; 2006. p. 401–17.
27. Ghneim GS, Viers JH, Chomel BB, et al. Use of a case-control study and geographic information systems to determine environmental and demographic risk factors for canine leptospirosis. Vet Res 2007;38(1):37–50.
28. Greenlee JJ, Alt DP, Bolin CA, et al. Experimental canine leptospirosis caused by leptospira interrogans serovars pomona and bratislava. AmJ Vet Res. 2005; 66(10):1816–22.
29. Baumann D, Flückiger M. Radiographic findings in the thorax of dogs with leptospiral infection. Vet Radiol Ultrasound 2001;42:305–7.
30. Stokes JE, Kaneene JB, Schall WD, et al. Prevalence of serum antibodies against six *Leptospira* serovars in healthy dogs. J Am Vet Med Assoc 2007;230(11):1657–64.
31. Forrest LJ, O'Brien RT, Tremelling MS, et al. Sonographic renal findings in 20 dogs with leptospirosis. Vet Radiol Ultrasound 1998;39(4):337–40.
32. Levett PN. Usefulness of serologic analysis as a predictor of the infecting serovar in patients with severe leptospirosis. Clin Infect Dis 2003;36(4):447–52.
33. Chandrasekaran S, Pankajalakshmi VV. Usefulness of dark field microscopy after differential centrifugation in the early diagnosis of leptospirosis in dog and its human contacts. Indian J Med Sci 1997;51:1–4.
34. Torten M, Shenberg E, Van der Hoeden J. The use of immunofluorescence in the diagnosis of human leptospirosis by a genus-specific antigen. J Infect Dis 1966; 116:537–43.
35. Bal AE, Gravekamp C, Hartskeerl RA, et al. Detection of leptospires in urine by PCR for early diagnosis of leptospirosis. J Clin Microbiol 1994;32:1894–8.
36. Merien F, Baranton G, Perolat P. Comparison of polymerase chain reaction with microagglutination test and culture for diagnosis of leptospirosis. J Infect Dis 1995;172:281–5.
37. Smythe LD, Smith IL, Smith GA, et al. A quantitative PCR (TaqMan) assay for pathogenic *Leptospira* spp. BMC Infect Dis 2002;2:13.
38. DeCaballero OL, et al. Low-stringency PCR with diagnostically useful primers for identification of *Leptospira* serovars. J Clin Microbiol 1994;32:1369–72.
39. Costa E, Lopes AA, Sacramento E, et al. Penicillin at the late stage of leptospirosis: a randomized controlled trial. Rev Inst Med Trop Sao Paulo 2003;45(3): 141–5.
40. Chandler AM, Goldstein RE. Assessing renal colonization in non-vaccinated dogs and in dogs 15 months after receiving a multi-serovar bacterin based vaccine, all experimentally infected with leptospira kirschneri serovar grippotyphosa [abstract]. In: Forum of the American College of Veterinary Internal Medicine, 2010
41. Moore GE, Guptill LF, Ward MP. Adverse events diagnosed within three days of vaccine administration in dogs. J Am Vet Med Assoc 2005;227(7):1102–8.

Lyme Borreliosis in Dogs and Cats: Background, Diagnosis, Treatment and Prevention of Infections with *Borrelia burgdorferi* sensu stricto

Inke Krupka, Dr Med Vet, Reinhard K. Straubinger, PhD*

KEYWORDS

• Dog • Lyme borreliosis • Lyme disease • Borrelia • Tick

INSIGHTS: MICROBIOLOGY, TAXONOMY, NATURAL HABITATS, AND TRANSMISSION CYCLE

The borrelia that cause Lyme borreliosis (LB) are approximately 25 μm long and only 0.2 μm in diameter, which makes the organisms nearly invisible when bright-field microscopy is used for detection. Therefore, dark-field microscopy is used for visualization. Spirochetes are motile in fluids and most likely body tissues. According to their natural doubling time of approximately 12 hours, they grow slowly in liquid and semisolid cultures at 33°C (**Fig. 1**). Their protoplasmatic cylinder contains cell organelles and is enclosed by a double-layer membrane. Seven to 11 periplasmatic endoflagella, which originate in basal bodies at both cell poles, form a rigid axial rod, around which the protoplasmatic cylinder is wound. The endoflagella undergo a structure variation that enables the bacteria to move in a wavelike motion. The periplasmatic environment is surrounded by a second cell membrane that contains a variety of outer membrane proteins. Like in many other bacteria, a mucous, amorphous layer encloses the outer membrane. Its function is still unclear, but a role in binding components of the

Bacteriology and Mycology, Institute for Infectious Diseases and Zoonoses, Department of Veterinary Sciences, Ludwig-Maximilians-University, Veterinärstraße 13, 80539 Munich, Germany
* Corresponding author.
E-mail address: R.Straubinger@lmu.de

Vet Clin Small Anim 40 (2010) 1103–1119
doi:10.1016/j.cvsm.2010.07.011
0195-5616/10/$ – see front matter © 2010 Elsevier Inc. All rights reserved.

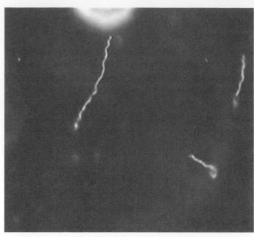

Fig. 1. *B burgdorferi* sensu stricto visualized by dark-field microscopy. (*Courtesy of* Dr Reinhard K. Straubinger, PhD, Germany.)

surrounding environment such as the host's complement factor H or plasminogen via special receptors is discussed.[1] Unlike leptospira, borrelia have a low tenacity and cannot survive in the environment outside the tick, mammalian, or avian host, as a result of their dependency on essential metabolic products from the host and their specific temperature requirements (eg, 30–42°C).

Borrelia belong to the genus *Borrelia* within the family Spirochaetaceae, which also includes the genera *Treponema*, *Cristispira* and *Spirochaeta*. The Spirochaetaceae are subordinated in the order of *Spirochaetales*, together with the families Leptospiraceae, Brachyspiraceae and Brevinemaceae. The genus *Borrelia* is heterogeneous and includes a complex of species that can be functionally summarized as relapsing-fever borrelia, such as *B recurrentis* (endemic louse-borne relapsing fever in humans), *B lonestari* (southern tick-associated rash illness in humans) and *B anserina* (avian spirochetosis in poultry). All borrelia that are transmitted by *Ixodes* ticks and are associated with LB infections are functionally grouped in the *B burgdorferi* sensu lato complex, which currently comprises 15 species (**Table 1**). For several species in this group such as *B americana, B californiensis, B caroliniensis,*[2–4] which have recently been identified after isolation from ticks in North America, the pathogenicity in people or animals has not been proved so far. For the other species causing LB, worldwide distribution and the effect of the disease is a complicated issue. Since the first etiologic description of LB in 1983 by Willy Burgdorfer, in North America only the species *B burgdorferi* sensu stricto has been found to be pathologic in humans and in dogs.[5,6] In contrast, in central Europe, Scandinavia and parts of Asia, at least 3 species have been identified to cause clinical apparent LB in humans: *B burgdorferi* sensu stricto, *B garinii*, and *B afzelii*. The experimental proof that natural infection with *B afzelii* and *B garinii* occurs in dogs is still missing, but DNA of these species was found in naturally infected dogs.[7,8] Because transmitting ticks in Europe and Asia can simultaneously carry *B burgdorferi* sensu stricto, *B garinii*, and *B afzelii* as well as *B valaisiana*, *B spielmanii*, and *B lusitaniae*, species-specific diagnosis in Europe is challenging. The infection rates of ticks is 34.4% for *B afzelii*, 25.1% for *B garinii*, 22.0% for *B burgdorferi* sensu stricto, 12.7% for *B valaisiana*, and 5.9% for *B spielmanii*[9] in southern Germany. *B spielmanii* and *B lusitaniae* have also been

Table 1
Species of the *Borrelia burgdorferi* sensu lato complex

Species	Geographic Distribution
B burgdorferi sensu stricto	North America, Europe
B garinii	Europe, Asia
B afzelii	Europe, Asia
B valaisiana	Europe, Asia
B spielmanii	Europe
B lusitaniae	Europe, North Africa
B andersonii	North America
B bissettii	North America, Europe
B tanukii	Asia
B turdii	Europe, Asia
B japonica	Asia (Japan)
B sinica	Asia
B californiensis sp. nov.	North America (west)
B carolinensis sp. nov.	North America (south-east)
B americana sp. nov.	North America (south-east, west)

isolated from skin lesions found on human patients and thus are believed to be causative agents of LB. Commonly, the worldwide distribution of LB follows endemic areas of ticks: climatic zones of moderate humidity and temperature and a vegetation of mixed to deciduous forests and brushwoods. These are the optimal living conditions for the transmitting arthropod vector: hard-shelled ticks of the genus *Ixodes*. In North America, they are represented mainly by 3 different species: *I scapularis* (midwestern, north- to south-eastern parts of the United States), formerly named *Ixodes dammini*; *I pacificus* and *I neotomae* (western and central states of the United States). In Europe (central, northern, and western parts of the continent), *I ricinus* is the main vector for *B burgdorferi* sensu lato species; in eastern parts of Europe and Asia *I persulcatus* can transmit different borrelia species. Following the different vegetation and climatic zones, the infection rate of the ticks is regionally distinct. For example, in North America, the infection rate of *I scapularis* can reach up to 50% in adult ticks.[10] Generally, the infection rate of ixodid ticks increases with the life cycle of the vector (~10% in nymphs, ~20% in adults) and can reach up to 75% in central Europe.[11]

Ticks become infected by feeding on reservoir hosts during their 2- to 3-year life cycle. Tick larvae feed on small mammals such as rodents, moles, squirrels, birds, or even lizards during the first year of their life. After overwintering, the larvae molt into nymphs and subsequently feed on larger mammals such as deer, elks, or dogs, cats, humans, and horses. In this stage, nymphs are still only 2 to 3 mm in diameter can easily be overseen on humans or animals, which predestines them as an important and dangerous source of infection. During tick feeding, naive hosts can become infected via preinfected nymphs; noninfected nymphs can become infected with borrelia by feeding in close proximity to infected ticks.[12] During the autumn of the same year, nymphs molt into adults. The mature female ticks take their last blood meal on large mammalian hosts such as deer, dogs, humans, or horses. After insemination during this feeding on hosts by the male tick and after completion of the blood meal, the female leaves the host by dropping to the ground and lays around 3000 eggs in semi-solid soil. Transovarial infection of the eggs is uncommon and was documented only in single cases,[13] which enforces the denotation of wild reservoir hosts as the source of infection.

TRANSMISSION BETWEEN HOSTS

Almost the only form of natural transmission to a vertebrate host is by the bite of an infected tick, although experimental data have affirmed the presence of DNA and antibodies in puppies born to a bitch that was needle-inoculated and infected with borrelia before gestation. The puppies did not receive colostrum and milk from their mother, which points to the possibility of diaplacentar transmission.[14] However, vertical and horizontal transfer of borrelia was not traceable when dogs were infected via tick bites.[15,16]

HOW TO LEAVE THE TICK

During the first 12 to 24 hours after the tick bite, borrelia organisms residing in the tick's midgut are not transmitted to the vertebrate host. During this time, the spirochetes undergo a complex process in outer surface remodeling to survive later in the immunocompetent mammalian or avian host. One activator of this process is most likely the increase of temperature, that the tick experiences during the blood meal in close contact with the host's skin. The virulence of the borrelia depends to a certain extent on the switch of their outer surface proteins (Osp) from OspA to OspC.[17] Not all spirochetes in a tick complete the restructuring process. Some still express OspA and it was shown that OspA-presenting bacteria cannot withstand the host's immune response. In contrast, the OspC protein is variable.[18,19] OspC was shown to be essential for the spirochetes to penetrate the tick's midgut and to establish an infection in the vertebrate host.[20,21] Another cofactor, tick salivary protein 15 (Salp15) binds to OspC-coated borrelia in the tick and covers the spirochetes and protects against attacks of the immune system[22] about 24 to 48 hours after the initial tick bite.[19,23]

HOW TO SURVIVE IN THE VERTEBRATE HOST

How borrelia disseminate through the mammalian host is still under discussion. One hypothesis postulates that borrelia disseminate via the bloodstream through the body and can survive in the blood, as shown in blood bank conditions,[24] and can colonize distant body sites by leaving the blood stream at various body sites. The other hypothesis suggests that blood, with its cellular and soluble immunologic components, is a hostile environment, forcing borrelia to migrate through tissue and settle in collagen-rich tissues (eg, joint capsules, skin, perineurium) where they can proliferate and survive for years. In this context it was shown that borrelia can generally be found in the extracellular matrix of infected dogs,[25] and it is known that borrelia are dependent on N-acetyl-glucosamine, which is a prerequisite to produce collagen.[26] This could explain the tropism to skin and the pathologic lesions found in and around collagen-rich tissues. To migrate actively through the host's body, borrelia are also able to bind plasminogen and plasminogen activator, which help to digest the extracellular matrix of body tissues.[27] Because borreliae do not belong to the group of gram-negative bacteria, they do not produce and contain typical lipopolysaccharides.[28] Nevertheless, spirochetal cells present a variety of proteins and lipoproteins on their surface, such as the OspC as mentioned earlier. To evade efficiently the host's immune response, spirochetes produce another outer membrane lipoprotein called VlsE (variable major protein-like sequence, expressed). The amino acid sequence of the structure varies rapidly within days after infection.[29] It was shown that borrelial clones, which are not able to change the VlsE sequence as quickly as other clones, are preferentially recognized and killed by the immune system.[30] The production of specific antibodies against swiftly changing antigenic variants occurs much slower. Antibodies produced against former VlsE variants cannot bind to the new VlsE epitopes, and consequently cannot neutralize the borrelial cell. VlsE is not expressed in borrelia residing in ticks.[31,32] This predestines VlsE and its constant regions (eg, IR6 or C6 peptide) as a specific diagnostic tool to detect antibodies against metabolic active LB spirochetes, especially in humans and dogs.[33] Furthermore, borrelia can probably survive the host's immune response by transforming their screwlike body into a round vesicle within a few minutes. Perhaps this feature allows them to survive unfavorable conditions exploiting a minimized cell metabolism.[34]

THE EFFECT OF THE HOST'S IMMUNE RESPONSE

Typically, LB is seen as a subclinical or intermitting acute clinical disease and may progress to a chronic illness. One reason for this development may be that LB spirochetes cannot be eliminated effectively by the host's immune response and antibodies that are formed during infection. The reasons for this ineffectiveness are complex immune evasion mechanisms of the typically extracellularly living borrelia. After the spirochetes have entered the host's tissues via a tick bite and saliva, the mediators of the innate immune response, such as granulocytes and macrophages, migrate to the site of inoculation and engage in the elimination of spirochetes via phagocytosis[35,36] or extracellular killing by releasing oxidative radicals. This process occurs hours to days after infection. These quick, but unspecific inflammatory responses may induce postinfection symptoms in the form of an *erythema migrans*, a reddish circular skin rash around the tick bite found in humans and rabbits. However, this local killing of borrelia is not exhaustive and does not eliminate the infection effectively.[36] Consequently, spirochetes continue to disseminate and induce multisystemic inflammatory responses that are caused by the aggressive content of granula produced by polymorphonuclear neutrophiles (PMN).

The production of specific antibodies starts late after the initial infection compared with other bacterial infections. Immumoglobulin (Ig) M antibody levels begin to increase 2 to 4 weeks after the infection, and detectable IgG antibodies can be found about 4 to 6 weeks after infection.[37] In experimentally infected beagles, peak levels of IgG were found approximately 90 days after tick exposure.[16] As mentioned earlier, antibodies induced by infection do not induce a protective immunity in people or dogs.

In the late and chronic stage of the disease, massive infiltrates of T lymphocytes can be found in synovial joints and sometimes around the perineurium. Those reactions are induced by cytokines such as interleukin (IL)-8.[38] However, many other cytokines (eg, IL-10 and IL-4) are involved in the pathogenesis of LB and it was shown that LB bacteria can suppress the release of some of these factors.[39] In this way, the immune response is modified into a proinflammatory or antibody-inducing T-cell response. In addition, the role of an autoimmune response during chronic Lyme arthritis in humans with a special type of cell surface molecules (MHC II HLA-DR4) is still under discussion.[40] As a result, the lesions observed during LB are less the result of direct tissue damage induced by borrelia and more the consequences seen after an exuberant effect of an overwhelmed immune system.

CLINICAL LB IN DOGS

Unlike human LB, the clinical phases of the disease in dogs cannot be divided clearly into 3 stages. Although experimentally infected monkeys showed clinical signs similar to those seen in humans, the dog nevertheless seems to be the most susceptible domestic animal, and serves as a sentinel and an appropriate animal model to investigate human LB.

In most cases the exact time point of infection via tick bite cannot be determined in dogs, because the feeding tick (adults or nymphs) are overlooked by the owner. It is commonly accepted that not all infected individuals continue to develop clinically apparent disease. In experimentally induced infections, up to 75% of all infected dogs developed disease.[15] No broad epidemiologic data are available so far on clinical disease in naturally infected dogs. Contrary to common beliefs, the presence of serum antibodies does not correlate with clinical signs and many infected dogs seroconvert and stay asymptomatic.[10]

Days to Weeks After Initial Infection

The first signs of clinical disease are unspecific and do not develop in all dogs; acute signs can be fever, general malaise, lameness, and swelling of local lymph nodes.[41] This stage is often overlooked or is not followed by the owner, because these first symptoms generally disappear after a few days. Erythema migrans, which can be found in many humans, has not been described in dogs; but a small, reddish lesion approximately 1 cm in diameter can be found around the tick bite. This reaction, an inflammatory response to the tick bite, disappears within days after removal of the tick.

Weeks to Months After Initial Infection

Joints and lameness

With the dissemination of the spirochetes into the skin, joints, and connective tissues, local inflammatory reactions can cause pain, swelling, and lameness. Dogs became lame 2 to 6 months after experimentally induced infections.[41] Severe lameness lasted for 2 to 5 days as a mono- or oligoarthritis. It was recognized first at the site of tick infestation, which reinforces the centrifugal spread of bacteria through the body.[41] The lameness was described as intermittent limping and sometimes recurred 2 to 3 weeks later in the same limb or another limb. In addition, an increased level of synovial fluid was noted with cell counts in the joint cavity ranging between 3000 and 100,000 cells/μL. In naturally infected dogs, recurrence of lameness associated with fatigue, moderate increase in body temperature, and pain in movements walking up or down stairs was described. An interesting aspect is the potential role of arthropathy caused by ruptured cruciate ligaments; in dogs living in endemic areas that were affected with this syndrome, more bacterial DNA was found in synovial biopsies.[42] However, rupture of the cruciate ligament is still an important differential diagnosis for Lyme arthritis.

Kidney involvement and breed predisposition for disease

In natural infected dogs, glomerulonephritis with protein loss was described for certain breeds.[43] Fatal and progressive renal disease including peripheral edema, azotemia, uremia, proteinuria, and effusion into body cavities was often associated with emesis. Lethargy was also documented in the study, in which 49 cases were further analyzed; disease was lethal or resulted in euthanasia for all dogs after 1 day to 8 weeks after onset.[44] Even though specific antibodies against *B burgdorferi* were detectable in some dogs, no viable bacteria were cultivated from renal tissue. Most dogs were Labrador retrievers or golden retrievers. Renal disease in conjunction with suspected LB was also described in Bernese mountain dogs. High antibody levels not associated with clinical disease are often reported in this breed in publications from

Switzerland.[45,46] In these studies, 58% of all Bernese mountain dogs tested were seropositive, whereas only 5% of dogs from other large-sized breeds developed antibodies against *B burgdorferi* sensu lato. However, a predisposition of these breeds for developing renal disease after infection with *B burgdorferi* sensu lato was not proved under experimental conditions.

Nerves, meninges, and inflammation

During infection, humans infrequently suffer from neuropathologic signs resulting from aseptic meningitis or a so-called Bannwarth syndrome.[47,48] Neurologic symptoms are often associated with infections with *B garinii* in European patients,[49] but this has not been confirmed in dogs. Neuropathologic findings in experimentally infected dogs were described as an asymptomatic encephalitis, mild perineuritis, or meningitis only.[25]

Other manifestations

A case study reporting myocarditis and cardiac arrhythmia in a dog was published during the early days of LB, but spirochetes could not be detected in cardiac tissue.[50] In many cases, LB is considered based on speculation. In a serologic study on dogs from Germany, which analyzed the preliminary clinical reports of 512 dog owners and veterinarians, only 6.7% of the dogs with suspected LB carried specific antibodies against *B burgdorferi* sensu lato; 33.3% of all seronegative dogs showed typical symptoms of LB such as lameness and fever (Inke Krupka, unpublished data, 2009).

The Potential Effects of Coinfection with Anaplasma Phagocytophilum

The rickettsial bacterium *Anaplasma phagocytophilum* is often found in ixodid ticks that carry *B burgdorferi* and it was shown that dogs can develop antibodies against *B burgdorferi* and *A phagocytophilum* concurrently.[51] Dogs living in LB-endemic areas of the United States and concurrently carrying antibodies against *B burgdorferi* and *A phagocytophilum* were more prone to show clinical signs than dogs with single infections.[52] Especially when thrombocytopenia, fatigue, and lameness occur, a potential infection with *A phagocytophilum* should be considered.[53]

LB IN CATS

Cats also suffer from tick bites and are hosts for *Ixodes* ticks. However, no case of a cat naturally infected with clinical LB has been described so far. Nevertheless, experimental infections via spirochete inoculation different from tick exposure resulted in short-lived bacteremia. If the cats were exposed to tick bites, they developed lameness and multilocalized inflammations such as arthritis or meningitis.[54] Cats also developed measurable antibody responses. In northern parts of the United States, where LB is endemic, 13% to 47% of cats were found to be seropositive.[55] It still is unclear why cats do not react as sensitively to a borrelial infection as dogs, but it is hypothesized that they are not as susceptible to the dissemination of the spirochetes or that their immune response can neutralize the bacteria before clinical illness occurs.

CLINICAL AND LABORATORY DIAGNOSIS

The definitive diagnosis of LB is still a difficult and often long process resulting in many differential diagnoses in human and in veterinary medicine, because no specific all-encompassing test for LB is available. The great public interest in the disease, over interpretation, and less specific laboratory tests can result in false-positive diagnoses. On the other hand, the spirochete is difficult to detect and subclinical infections are common. In addition, the late immunologic antibody response and late clinical manifestations often delay diagnosis and efficient treatment. To substantiate the diagnosis of LB, 4 criteria should be checked carefully:

1. Are the clinical signs seen in the patient associated with (typical for) LB?
2. Are specific antibodies against *B burgdorferi* detectable (vaccination needs to be considered)?
3. Does the patient improve substantially after an appropriate antibiotic therapy is applied?
4. Does the patient live in an endemic area for LB and is there a real risk of exposure to *Ixodes* spp ticks?

Laboratory Findings

Regarding laboratory findings, no specific pathognomonic parameters exist. Cell count may be increased in joint fluid and cerebrospinal fluid (CSF). PMN is the predominant cell type found during inflammation. In case of renal involvement, urine parameters may point to uremia as described earlier.

Serologic Testing

The indirect detection of *B burgdorferi* by detecting specific antibodies in blood or blood serum has become an important tool in diagnosing LB. However, the direct detection methods such as culture or microscopy are time consuming and are often not sensitive enough, because the bacterial burden in tissue samples or body fluids is generally low. It cannot be emphasized enough that the detection of specific antibodies against *B burgdorferi* does not necessarily correlate with the presence of clinical disease, especially in endemic areas or in dogs that have been treated with antibiotics previously. In addition, IgG levels are generally not detectable during the first 4 weeks after tick exposure and spirochete infection. Generally, a detectable antibody level indicates immunologic contact with borrelial antigens. Many different assays are available as rapid tests for use in veterinary practice or as more sophisticated laboratory tests. The value of some serologic tests is often over estimated, because many test methods are not very specific and cross-reactions to other bacterial antigens occur.[56] In the past years, two-tiered test methods have been developed, including infection-specific tests using recombinant antigens. Unfortunately, test results can vary according to the test method applied and also among laboratories. Even day-to-day variation in the same laboratory is possible, when the same sample is tested repeatedly.

One of the first established serologic methods for LB testing was the indirect immunofluorescent antibody test. Because the specificity of the test is low and cross-reactive antibodies often lead to false-positive results, this method cannot be recommended, especially when used as a single test.

ENZYME-LINKED IMMUNOSORBENT ASSAY AND IMMUNOBLOTTING: A TWO-TIERED TEST SYSTEM

This two-tiered laboratory test is the most common assay for LB used today and is the method of choice for LB serodiagnosis.[57] It consists of 2 components: a highly sensitive screening method based on an enzyme-linked immunosorbent assay (ELISA) to filter out negative samples with high fidelity. Equivocal samples require confirmation. Immunoblotting (Western blotting) is used in a second step to characterize positive samples further or to differentiate between infected or vaccinated animals. Generally, these tests can be performed with whole-cell preparations of borrelial antigens or with recombinant antigen from borrelia. The benefit of whole-cell preparations is their intrinsic high sensitivity; cross-reactivity with nonspecific antibodies occurs frequently. The use of recombinant proteins, especially in commercial tests, has increased in recent years because these tests are well standardized.

Methods based on ELISA techniques allow the detection of IgM and/or IgG subclasses. In veterinary medicine, IgM detection is not common or recommended, because clinical signs develop weeks after tick exposure when detectable IgG are already present. As mentioned earlier, experimentally infected dogs produced detectable antibody levels 4 to 6 weeks after exposure (IgG detection with whole-cell preparation).[15,58] These IgG antibodies persisted for years; even after successful antibiotic treatment these antibodies were detectable for years in otherwise healthy individuals.

Immunoblotting is more time consuming and more difficult to interpret than other serologic detection methods; for this reason it is generally not used as a single test. Immunoblots help to make a final decision whether ELISA-positive samples are considered positive for antibodies specific to *B burgdorferi* or not. Visualized antibody-antigen-signals are specific in size (kilodalton, kDa) and their location on the Western blot depends on the borrelia species used for the test. In North America, the use of antigens derived from *B burgdorferi* sensu stricto is common, whereas in Europe, *B afzelii* is the recommended species.[59,60] Using immunoblotting, the differentiation between infection- and vaccination-specific antibodies or both in the same sample is possible (**Fig. 2**). An overview of the most important proteins of *B burgdorferi*, which can be seen on an immunoblot incubated with serum from dogs, is given in **Table 2**. A signal at 31 kDa (OspA) occurs when antibodies from vaccinated dogs bind to this antigen. This signal is rarely seen in naturally infected dogs.[61]

TEST SYSTEMS BASED ON THE INVARIABLE REGION 6 (IR$_6$) OF VLSE

According to current knowledge, the highly variable surface protein, VlsE, is exclusively expressed in the mammalian host (see section on How to survive in the vertebrate host). The invariable region (IR$_6$), and even a shorter peptide sequence of IR$_6$ called C$_6$ were found to have high potential as specific antigenic components in serologic test systems. This was shown by evaluating sera from infected humans, dogs, monkeys, and mice.[33] VlsE and IR$_6$ are highly conserved among genospecies of the *B burgdorferi* sensu lato complex.[62] Based on the amino acid sequence of IR$_6$, a 25-mer synthetic analogue C$_6$ peptide was developed and used as a successful ELISA tool to specify the clinical effect of immune responses against *B burgdorferi* in human infections.[63] C$_6$ antibodies were detectable even during the early phase of the infection. Furthermore, no cross-reactivities against vaccination-specific OspA antibodies were found. Further studies proved this characteristic by testing sera of vaccinated dogs using a C$_6$ peptide–coated ELISA.[64,65] Moreover, in experimentally infected dogs C$_6$-specific IgG antibodies appeared 3 weeks after infection, almost 1 week earlier than antibodies detected with ELISA-based whole-cell preparations.[65] In addition, another benefit became clear when testing sera of humans and dogs before and after antibiotic treatment. Contrary to antibodies against whole-cell components, levels of C$_6$ antibodies decreased and remained so a few months after treatment.[66] However, in animals with low C$_6$ antibody levels before treatment, the decrease was minimal after treatment.[67] A commercial C$_6$ ELISA is available for dogs to document treatment success approximately 4 to 6 months after therapy (C$_6$ Quant ELISA, IDEXX Laboratories Inc, ME, USA). Despite their high specificity

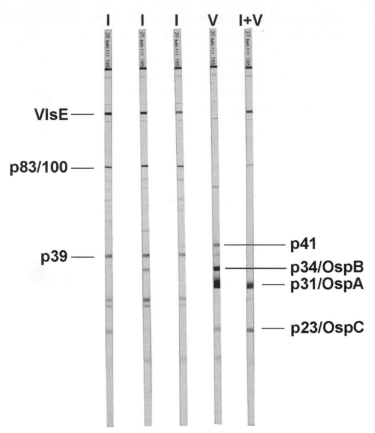

Fig. 2. Immunoblot developed with canine sera on whole-cell lysate-antigen and recombinant VlsE (*B afzelii*+VlsE Eco Blot, Genzyme Virotech, Germany). I, experimentally infected dog (*B burgdorferi* sensu stricto); V, experimentally vaccinated dog (lysate vaccine); I+V, infected and vaccinated dog (lysate vaccine). (*Courtesy of* Dr Inke Krupka, Germany.)

for borrelial contact, C_6 antibodies do not necessarily correlate with clinical signs in dogs and false-positive results may result from maternal antibodies in puppies born to infected bitches.[68] Treatment of C_6-positive dogs independent of the presence of illness should be considered carefully. The use of C_6 antibody testing in veterinary practice is recommended to clarify whether lameness seen in patients is the result of an infection with *B burgdorferi* or by other tick-transmitted organisms such as *A phagocytophilum*.

Direct Detection of B Burgdorferi

LB spirochetes in tissue samples (eg, skin biopsy samples), blood, or synovial fluids need up to 6 weeks for bacterial growth when transferred into special liquid medium (eg, BSK-II, Babour-Stoenner-Kelley medium). Despite the high specificity, sensitivity of culture can be low because spirochetes are often present at low numbers in tissues. Chances of detection success are higher if a 4- to 6-mm skin biopsy punch sample is collected near the site of the assumed tick bite. The samples need to be handled sterilely to reduce the risk of medium contamination.

Table 2
Protein bands that can be seen on a Western blot specific for *Borrelia burgdorferi*

Protein Band	Size (kDa)	Specificity in Serology/Function in Borrelial Cells
p14	14	Highly specific, unknown function
p17	17	Highly specific, outer surface protein
p21	21	Highly specific, unknown function
OspC	21–23	Highly specific, outer surface protein
p30	30	Highly specific, unknown function
OspA	31–33	Highly specific, outer surface protein
OspB	34–36	Moderately specific, outer surface protein
p39 (BmpA)	39	Moderately specific, membrane protein
p41	41	Less specific, cross-reactive with antibodies against other bacteria, flagellin
p43	43	Highly specific, unknown function
p58	58	Highly specific, unknown function
p66	66	Highly specific, membrane-associated protein
p60, p75	60–75	Less specific, cross-reactive antibodies with antibodies against other bacteria; heat shock proteins
p83–p100	83–100	Highly specific, associated with the protoplasmatic membrane or the flagella

The polymerase chain reaction (PCR) amplifies borrelial DNA and can produce results quickly in a few hours. Contrary to culture, the PCR cannot distinguish between viable and dead spirochetes,[5] and the chance to find borrelia in naturally infected dogs is low, again because of low bacterial burdens. The effect of false-negative results consequently is high. This method is recommended for skin or synovial tissue rather than body fluids such as blood or CSF[69] because the spirochetes are predominantly present in tissue of persistently infected individuals. The method can lead to misinterpretation if it is used as a single standard diagnostic tool without taking into account serologic data and clinical signs. Nevertheless, PCR can be a helpful scientific tool for the detection and differentiation of borrelial species or strains in an epidemiologic survey.

THERAPY
Antimicrobial Therapy

Contrary to LB in humans, the time of infection cannot be pinpointed in most animals, and most cases that the veterinarian decides to treat are in a phase in which the spirochetes have already disseminated into various tissues. Because the success rate of antimicrobial treatment is higher during the early stages of the disease, treatment should be initiated as early as possible. In these cases, antibody levels may decrease and lameness or other disorders may be reduced or disappear completely within 1 to 3 days after initiation of treatment.[16] The question of whether dogs (or cats) should be treated when specific antibodies are detected in the absence of clinical signs is controversial.[10,70,71] We believe that only clinically apparent individuals should be treated. Generally, treatment is recommended for a period of 28 to 30 days.

Borrelia organisms are sensitive to tetracyclines (doxycycline), amoxicillin, azithromycin, and cephalosporines. The most commonly used drug is doxycycline, because it can be given orally and is not expensive. In addition, possible coinfections with

Anaplasma and *Ehrlichia* species can be treated. Amoxicillin is preferred for sensitive and growing individuals. Encephalitis in humans caused by borrelia is treated with cephalosporines, because these drugs penetrate the blood-brain barrier more efficiently.[72] Treatment regimens are listed in **Table 3** and concur with other published recommendations.[10,16] In chronic cases, borreliae are not eliminated completely with a single course of treatment. This was shown in experimentally infected dogs.[16] As a result, clinical lameness or other signs may reoccur and treatment needs to be repeated.

Prevention with Antibiotics

This method is uncommon in veterinary medicine, because it is expensive and the time of tick infestation is unknown in most cases.

Therapy with Nonsteroidal and Steroidal Antiinflammatory Drugs

Pain management with nonsteroidal drugs can be helpful, especially for bouts of severe lameness and arthritic disorders despite the risk of gastroenteric irritation. Glucocorticoids should be given only in doses that are not immunosuppressive and in combination with antibiotics.

PROPHYLAXIS
Vaccination

A variety of vaccines is available worldwide for prevention of LB in dogs. The mode of prevention is unique, because antibodies induced by vaccination do not fight the borrelia in the dog but in the tick. Vaccine-induced OspA-specific antibodies circulate in the dog's blood, and are ingested by the tick via the blood meal. OspA antibodies can bind to the OspA-expressing borrelia in the tick, prevent their migration to the salivary glands and reduce their growth in the tick.[73] If borreliae have already infected the host, the bacteria are not affected by OspA antibodies, because these borreliae have switched completely to OspC/VlsE surface expression, and a seroconversion as a result of OspA via natural infection is uncommon in practice.[74] Vaccination must induce high antibody levels in the dog before tick exposure, and the spirochete transfer from ticks to dogs is prevented only during phases with high OspA antibody levels. Hence, frequent revaccination is essential.

Whole-cell lysate and recombinant OspA vaccines are currently available in the United States. They are based on *B burgdorferi* sensu stricto proteins.[10] In Europe, lysate vaccines produced with *B burgdorferi* sensu stricto or with *B garinii* and *B afzelii* are on the market. Again, the European situation is more complicated as more

Table 3
Antimicrobial agents and therapy regimes available for LB

Agent	Duration (days)	Interval (times daily)	Route	Dose
Doxycycline	30	1–2	po	10 mg/kg
Amoxicillin	30	3	po	20 mg/kg
Azithromycin	10–20	1	po	25 mg/kg
Penicillin G	14–30	3	iv	22,000 U/kg
Cefotaxime	14–30	3	iv	20 mg/kg
Ceftriaxone	14–30	1	iv or sc	25 mg/kg

Abbreviations: iv, intravenous; po, per os; sc, subcutaneous.

pathogenic species are present in the ticks and complete cross-reactivity of the vaccine-induced antibodies is not documented.[58]

Vaccination schedules vary according to the provider and the vaccine. Initially, 2 immunizations are given 3 to 4 weeks apart. It is recommended to repeat vaccination 6 months later and again another 6 months later (in total 1 year after vaccination was initiated). From then on, annual revaccination is sufficient to sustain protective OspA antibody levels.[58]

In general, prevention against *B burgdorferi* infection via vaccination only is not recommended. Tick control is an important part of prophylaxis and the daily removal of ticks by the owner is essential, especially in endemic areas. The decision whether to vaccinate or not should always be based on careful consideration of individual behavior and circumstances, which include geographic location, outdoor activities, and risk of tick infestation.

Tick Prevention

Topical application of repellents or acaricides onto dogs to prevent tick infestation is effective. Several drugs and formulations are available, including spot-ons, powders, sprays, solutions, collars, and shampoos. If combined with daily tick removal, this method can be very effective. However, repellents that contain permethrin must not be used on cats because of its toxic effects on this species. Other drugs contain triazapentadienes (Amitraz) or phenylpyrazoles (Fipronil).

SUMMARY

Three fundamental elements (mechanical tick removal, tick prevention based on repellents or acaricides, immunization with vaccines against LB) prevent infection with *B burgdorferi* in most cases. If infection with *B burgdorferi* is nonetheless suspected, many differential diagnoses need to be considered, because no pathognomonic clinical sign is expressed during disease and no specific diagnostic test exists to reveal clinical LB. However, when clinical signs are present but ambiguous, the use of highly specific serodiagnostic tests can help to decide whether treatment is necessary.

REFERENCES

1. Haupt K, Kraiczy P, Wallich R, et al. Binding of human factor H-related protein I to serum-resistant *Borrelia burgdorferi* is mediated by borrelial complement regulator-acquiring surface proteins. J Infect Dis 2007;196(1):124–33.
2. Rudenko N, Golovchenko M, Grubhoffer L, et al. *Borrelia carolinensis* sp.nov. – a new (14th) member of *Borrelia burgdorferi* sensu lato complex from the southeastern United States. J Clin Microbiol 2009;47(1):134–41.
3. Rudenko N, Golovchenko M, Lin T, et al. Delineation of a new species of the *Borrelia burgdorferi* sensu lato complex, *Borrelia americana* sp. J Clin Microbiol 2009;47(12):3875–80.
4. Postic D, Garnier M, Baranton G. Multilocus sequence analysis of atypical *Borrelia burgdorferi* sensu lato isolates–description of *Borrelia californiensis* sp. nov., and genomospecies 1 and 2. Int J Med Microbiol 2007;297(4):263–71.
5. Steere AC. Lyme disease. N Engl J Med 2001;345(2):115–25.
6. Appel MJ. Lyme disease in dogs and cats. Compend Cont Educ Pract Vet 1990; 12:617–26.
7. Hovius KE, Stark LA, Bleumink-Pluym NM, et al. Presence and distribution of *Borrelia burgdorferi* sensu lato species in internal organs and skin of naturally

infected symptomatic and asymptomatic dogs, as detected by polymerase chain reaction. Vet Q 1999;21(2):54–8.

8. Speck S, Reiner B, Wittenbrink MM. Isolation of *Borrelia afzelii* from a dog. Vet Rec 2001;149(1):19–20.

9. Fingerle V, Schulte-Spechtel UC, Ruzic-Sabljic E, et al. Epidemiological aspects and molecular characterization of *Borrelia burgdorferi* s.l. from southern Germany with special respect to the new species *Borrelia spielmanii* sp. nov. Int J Med Microbiol 2008;298(3–4):279–90.

10. Greene CE, Straubinger RK. Borreliosis. In: Greene CE, editor. Infectious diseases of the dog and cat. 3rd edition. Philadelphia: WB Saunders Elsevier; 2006. p. 417–35.

11. Rauter C, Hartung T. Prevalence of *Borrelia burgdorferi* sensu lato genospecies in *Ixodes ricinus* ticks in Europe: a metaanalysis. Appl Environ Microbiol 2005; 71(11):7203–16.

12. Ogden NH, Nuttall PA, Randolph SE. Natural Lyme disease cycles maintained *via* sheep by co-feeding ticks. Parasitology 1997;11:5591–9.

13. Nefedova VV, Korenberg EI, Gorelova NB, et al. Studies on the transovarial transmission of *Borrelia burgdorferi* sensu lato in the taiga tick *Ixodes persulcatus*. Folia Parasitol (Praha) 2004;51(1):67–71.

14. Gustafson JM, Burgess EC, Wachal MD, et al. Intrauterine transmission of *Borrelia burgdorferi* in dogs. Am J Vet Res 1993;54(6):882–90.

15. Appel MJ, Allen S, Jacobson RH, et al. Experimental Lyme disease in dogs produces arthritis and persistent infection. J Infect Dis 1993;167:651–64.

16. Straubinger RK, Straubinger AF, Summers BA, et al. Status of *Borrelia burgdorferi* infection after antibiotic treatment and the effects of corticosteroids: an experimental study. J Infect Dis 2000;181(3):1069–81.

17. Schwan TG, Piesman J, Golde WT, et al. Induction of an outer surface protein on *Borrelia burgdorferi* during tick feeding. Proc Natl Acad Sci U S A 1995;92(7): 2909–13.

18. Wilske B, Busch U, Fingerle V, et al. Immunological and molecular variability of OspA and OspC. Implication for *Borrelia* vaccine development. Infection 1996; 24(2):208–12.

19. Ohnishi J, Piesman J, de Silva AM. Antigenic and genetic heterogeneity of *Borrelia burgdorferi* populations transmitted by ticks. Proc Natl Acad Sci U S A 2001; 98(2):670–5.

20. Grimm D, Tilly K, Byram R, et al. Outer-surface protein C of the Lyme disease spirochete: a protein induced in ticks for infection of mammals. Proc Natl Acad Sci U S A 2004;101(9):3142–7.

21. Templeton TJ. *Borrelia* outer membrane surface proteins and transmission through the tick. J Exp Med 2004;199(5):603–6.

22. Schuijt TJ, Hovius JW, van Burgel ND, et al. Salp15 inhibits the killing of serum sensitive *Borrelia burgdorferi* sensu lato isolates. Infect Immun 2008.

23. Piesman J, Dolan MC, Happ CM, et al. Duration of immunity to reinfection with tick-transmitted *Borrelia burgdorferi* in naturally infected mice. Infect Immun 1997;65(10):4043–7.

24. Nadelman RB, Sherer C, Mack L, et al. Survival of *Borrelia burgdorferi* in human blood stored under blood banking conditions. Transfusion 1990;30(4): 298–301.

25. Straubinger RK, Straubinger AF, Summers BA, et al. Clinical manifestations, pathogenesis, and effect of antibiotic treatment on Lyme borreliosis in dogs. Wien Klin Wochenschr 1998;110(24):874–81.

26. Fraser CM, Casjens S, Huang WM, et al. Genomic sequence of a Lyme disease spirochaete, *Borrelia burgdorferi*. Nature 1997;390(6660):580–6.
27. Klempner MS, Noring R, Epstein MP, et al. Binding of human plasminogen and urokinase-type plasminogen activator to the Lyme disease spirochete, *Borrelia burgdorferi*. J Infect Dis 1995;17:11258–65.
28. Takayama K, Rothenberg RJ, Barbour AG. Absence of lipopolysaccharide in the Lyme disease spirochete, *Borrelia burgdorferi*. Infect Immun 1987;55(9):2311–3.
29. Embers ME, Liang FT, Howell JK, et al. Antigenicity and recombination of VlsE, the antigenic variation protein of *Borrelia burgdorferi*, in rabbits, a host putatively resistant to long-term infection with this spirochete. FEMS Immunol Med Microbiol 2007;50(3):421–9.
30. Coutte L, Botkin DJ, Gao L, et al. Detailed analysis of sequence changes occurring during vlsE antigenic variation in the mouse model of *Borrelia burgdorferi* infection. PLoS Pathog 2009;5(2):e1000293.
31. Indest KJ, Howell JK, Jacobs MB, et al. Analysis of *Borrelia burgdorferi* vlsE gene expression and recombination in the tick vector. Infect Immun 2001;69(11): 7083–90.
32. Zhang JR, Norris SJ. Kinetics and in vivo induction of genetic variation of vlsE in *Borrelia burgdorferi*. Infect Immun 1998;66(8):3689–97.
33. Liang FT, Philipp MT. Analysis of antibody response to invariable regions of VlsE, the variable surface antigen of *Borrelia burgdorferi*. Infect Immun 1999;67(12): 6702–6.
34. Gruntar I, Malovrh T, Murgia R, et al. Conversion of *Borrelia garinii* cystic forms to motile spirochetes in vivo. APMIS 2001;109(5):383–8.
35. Lusitani D, Malawista SE, Montgomery RR. Calprotectin, an abundant cytosolic protein from human polymorphonuclear leukocytes, inhibits the growth of *Borrelia burgdorferi*. Infect Immun 2003;71(8):4711–6.
36. Montgomery RR, Nathanson MH, Malawista SE. Fc- and non-Fc-mediated phagocytosis of *Borrelia burgdorferi* by macrophages. J Infect Dis 1994;170: 890–3.
37. Craft JE, Grodzicki RL, Shrestha M, et al. The antibody response in Lyme disease. Yale J Biol Med 1984;57(4):561–5.
38. Straubinger RK, Straubinger AF, Harter L, et al. *Borrelia burgdorferi* migrates into joint capsules and causes an up-regulation of interleukin-8 in synovial membranes of dogs experimentally infected with ticks. Infect Immun 1997; 65(4):1273–85.
39. Lazarus JJ, Kay MA, McCarter AL, et al. Viable *Borrelia burgdorferi* enhances interleukin-10 production and suppresses activation of murine macrophages. Infect Immun 2008;76(3):1153–62.
40. Kalish RA, Leong JM, Steere AC. Association of treatment-resistant chronic Lyme arthritis with HLA-DR4 and antibody reactivity to OspA and OspB of *Borrelia burgdorferi*. Infect Immun 1993;612:774–9.
41. Straubinger RK, Summers BA, Chang YF, et al. Persistence of *Borrelia burgdorferi* in experimentally infected dogs after antibiotic treatment. J Clin Microbiol 1997;35(1):111–6.
42. Muir P, Oldenhoff WE, Hudson AP, et al. Detection of DNA from a range of bacterial species in the knee joints of dogs with inflammatory knee arthritis and associated degenerative anterior cruciate ligament rupture. Microb Pathog 2007; 42(2-3):47–55.
43. Grauer GF, Burgess EC, Cooley AJ, et al. Renal lesions associated with *Borrelia burgdorferi* infection in a dog. J Am Vet Med Assoc 1988;193(2):237–9.

44. Dambach DM, Smith CA, Lewis RM, et al. Morphologic, immunohistochemical, and ultrastructural characterization of a distinctive renal lesion in dogs putatively associated with *Borrelia burgdorferi* infection: 49 cases (1987–1992). Vet Pathol 1997;34:85–96.

45. Gerber B, Eichenberger S, Wittenbrink MM, et al. Increased prevalence of *Borrelia burgdorferi* infections in Bernese Mountain Dogs: a possible breed predisposition. BMC Vet Res 2007;3(1):15.

46. Gerber B, Eichenberger S, Haug K, et al. [The dilemma with Lyme borreliosis in the dog with particular consideration of "Lyme nephritis"]. Schweiz Arch Tierheilkd 2009;151(10):479–83 [in German].

47. Halperin JJ. Nervous system Lyme disease. Infect Dis Clin North Am 2008;22(2): 261–74.

48. Vianello M, Marchiori G, Giometto B. Multiple cranial nerve involvement in Bannwarth's syndrome. Neurol Sci 2008;29(2):109–12.

49. Pachner AR, Steiner I. Lyme neuroborreliosis: infection, immunity, and inflammation. Lancet Neurol 2007;6(6):544–52.

50. Levy SA, Duray PH. Complete heart block in a dog seropositive for *Borrelia burgdorferi*. J Vet Intern Med 1988;21:38–44.

51. Greig B, Armstrong PJ. Canine granulocytotropic anaplasmosis (A phagocytophilum). In: Greene CE, editor. Infectious diseases of the dog and cat. 3rd edition. Philadelphia: Saunders Elsevier; 2006. p. 219–24.

52. Bowman D, Little SE, Lorentzen L, et al. Prevalence and geographic distribution of *Dirofilaria immitis*, *Borrelia burgdorferi*, *Ehrlichia canis*, and *Anaplasma phagocytophilum* in dogs in the United States: results of a national clinic-based serologic survey. Vet Parasitol 2009;160(1–2):138–48.

53. Beall M, Chandrashekar R, Eberts M, et al. *Borrelia burgdorferi* and *Anaplasma phagocytophilum*: potential implications of co-infection on clinical presentation in the dog. J Vet Intern Med 2006;20(No.3):713–4.

54. Gibson MD, Omran MT, Young CR. Experimental feline Lyme borreliosis as a model for testing *Borrelia burgdorferi* vaccines. Adv Exp Med Biol 1995;38: 373–82.

55. Magnarelli LA, Bushmich SL, IJdo JW, et al. Seroprevalence of antibodies against *Borrelia burgdorferi* and *Anaplasma phagocytophilum* in cats. Am J Vet Res 2005;66(11):1895–9.

56. Bruckbauer HR, Preac-Mursic V, Fuchs R, et al. Cross-reactive proteins of *Borrelia burgdorferi*. Eur J Clin Microbiol Infect Dis 1992;11(3):224–32.

57. Steere AC, McHugh G, Damle N, et al. Prospective study of serologic tests for Lyme disease. Clin Infect Dis 2008;47(2):188–95.

58. Toepfer KH, Straubinger RK. Characterization of the humoral immune response in dogs after vaccination against the Lyme borreliosis agent A study with five commercial vaccines using two different vaccination schedules. Vaccine 2007; 25(2):314–26.

59. Hauser U, Lehnert G, Lobentanzer R, et al. Interpretation criteria for standardized Western blots for three European species of *Borrelia burgdorferi* sensu lato. J Clin Microbiol 1997;35(6):1433–44.

60. Hauser U, Lehnert G, Wilske B. Validity of interpretation criteria for standardized Western blots (immunoblots) for serodiagnosis of Lyme borreliosis based on sera collected throughout Europe. J Clin Microbiol 1999;37(7):2241–7.

61. Greene RT, Walker RL, Nicholson WL, et al. Immunoblot analysis of immunoglobulin G to the Lyme disease agent (*Borrelia burgdorferi*) in experimentally and naturally infected dogs. J Clin Microbiol 1988;26:648–53.

62. Liang FT, Aberer E, Cinco M, et al. Antigenic conservation of an immunodominant invariable region of the VlsE lipoprotein among European pathogenic genospecies of *Borrelia burgdorferi* SL. J Infect Dis 2000;182(5):1455–62.

63. Liang FT, Steere AC, Marques AR, et al. Sensitive and specific serodiagnosis of Lyme disease by enzyme-linked immunosorbent assay with a peptide based on an immunodominant conserved region of *Borrelia burgdorferi* vlsE. J Clin Microbiol 1999;37(12):3990–6.

64. Levy SA. Use of a C6 ELISA test to evaluate the efficacy of a whole-cell bacterin for the prevention of naturally transmitted canine *Borrelia burgdorferi* infection. Vet Ther 2002;3(4):420–4.

65. Liang FT, Jacobson RH, Straubinger RK, et al. Characterization of a *Borrelia burgdorferi* VlsE invariable region useful in canine Lyme disease serodiagnosis by enzyme-linked immunosorbent assay. J Clin Microbiol 2000;38(11):4160–6.

66. Philipp MT, Bowers LC, Fawcett PT, et al. Antibody response to IR6, a conserved immunodominant region of the VlsE lipoprotein, wanes rapidly after antibiotic treatment of *Borrelia burgdorferi* infection in experimental animals and in humans. J Infect Dis 2001;184(7):870–8.

67. Levy SA, O'Connor TP, Hanscom JL, et al. Quantitative measurement of C6 antibody following antibiotic treatment of *Borrelia burgdorferi* antibody positive nonclinical dogs. Clin Vaccine Immunol 2008;15(1):115–9.

68. Eschner AK. Effect of passive immunoglobulin transfer on results of diagnostic tests for antibodies against *Borrelia burgdorferi* in pups born to a seropositive dam. Vet Ther 2008;9(3):184–91.

69. Straubinger RK. PCR-Based quantification of *Borrelia burgdorferi* organisms in canine tissues over a 500-day postinfection period. J Clin Microbiol 2000;38(6):2191–9.

70. Littman MP. Canine borreliosis. Vet Clin North Am Small Anim Pract 2003;33(4):827–62.

71. Littman MP, Goldstein RE, Labato MA, et al. ACVIM small animal consensus statement on Lyme disease in dogs: diagnosis, treatment, and prevention. J Vet Intern Med 2006;20(2):422–34.

72. Logigian EL, Kaplan RF, Steere AC. Successful treatment of Lyme encephalopathy with intravenous ceftriaxone. J Infect Dis 1999;180(2):377–83.

73. de Silva AM, Fish D, Burkot TR, et al. OspA antibodies inhibit the acquisition of *Borrelia burgdorferi* by *Ixodes* ticks. Infect Immun 1997;65(8):3146–50.

74. de Silva AM, Telford SR III, Brunet LR, et al. *Borrelia burgdorferi* OspA is an arthropod-specific transmission-blocking Lyme disease vaccine. J Exp Med 1996;183(1):271–5.

Ehrlichiosis and Anaplasmosis in Dogs and Cats

Susan E. Little, DVM, PhD

KEYWORDS

- Canine ehrlichiosis • Canine anaplasmosis • Feline ehrlichiosis
- Feline anaplasmosis

In the time since canine ehrlichiosis due to *Ehrlichia canis* was first described in 1935,[1] and first recognized in the United States in 1962,[2] many key advances have been made in our understanding of the diversity of the rickettsial organisms responsible for ehrlichiosis and anaplasmosis in dogs and, occasionally, cats, the vectors capable of transmitting these agents, and the role these organisms play as both important veterinary pathogens and zoonotic disease agents. Despite considerable progress in the field, much remains to be learned regarding mechanisms contributing to pathogenesis, effective treatment modalities, and prevention strategies that best protect pet health. This review highlights current understanding of the transmission, diagnosis, and management of ehrlichiosis and anaplasmosis in dogs and cats.

CANINE EHRLICHIOSIS
Agents of Canine Ehrlichiosis

Ehrlichiosis in dogs may be caused by *Ehrlichia canis*, *Ehrlichia chaffeensis*, *Ehrlichia ewingii*, or coinfection with these and other tick-borne pathogens. *E canis* is the ehrlichiosis agent first described from dogs and continues to be an important pathogen of dogs worldwide, responsible for severe, life-threatening illness.[3] *E chaffeensis* is better known as the agent of human monocytotropic ehrlichiosis (HME) in the southern United States, but also infects dogs. Experimental infections suggest that *E chaffeensis* produces relatively mild disease in dogs.[4] However, when coinfection with other ehrlichial agents is present, dogs may be more severely affected.[5] *E ewingii*, first described from a dog with febrile illness in 1971,[6] has since been shown to infect and cause disease in both dogs and people.[7,8] Although *E canis* is considered the primary ehrlichiosis agent of dogs in North America and worldwide, both *E ewingii* and *E chaffeensis* appear to be more common in dogs than *E canis* in areas with high vector tick populations, such as the south-central United States.[9,10]

Department of Veterinary Pathobiology, Center for Veterinary Health Sciences, Oklahoma State University, Stillwater, OK 74078-2007, USA
E-mail address: susan.little@okstate.edu

Tick Vectors, Reservoir Hosts, and Routes of Transmission

Dogs serve as a key reservoir host for *E canis* and also as the maintenance host for the primary vector tick, *Rhipicephalus sanguineus* (**Fig. 1**). Immature stages of *R sanguineus* are infected when feeding on a rickettsemic dog and then maintain that infection transstadially, enabling transmission to occur when the tick feeds again as a nymph or an adult.[11] Adult *R sanguineus* have also been shown to be capable of transmitting *E canis* intrastadially, a route that may be important in outbreak situations, as male ticks have been shown to readily move between dogs as they intermittently feed and mate.[12,13] The maintenance cycle of *E canis* is particularly pernicious because *R sanguineus* populations can establish and survive inside homes and kennels, providing a near-constant source of infection to dogs in an infested environment.[14] Although *R sanguineus* is the most common vector associated with *E canis* worldwide, *Dermacentor variabilis* has also been shown experimentally to transmit this pathogen.[15]

By contrast, *E chaffeensis* is maintained in nature in a cycle involving white-tailed deer as primary reservoir host and lone star ticks, *Amblyomma americanum* (see **Fig. 1**), as primary vector.[16] Dogs become infected when fed on by an infected nymph or adult *A americanum*, and infection of dogs and coyotes with *E chaffeensis* is common in areas with high *A americanum* populations.[17,18] Limited data from focal outbreaks suggest other secondary vectors, such as *D variabilis* and *R sanguineus*, may also be infected with and able to transmit *E chaffeensis* to dogs.[19–21] *A americanum* is also the primary vector tick for *E ewingii*.[22,23] Both dogs and deer have been shown to harbor *E ewingii* infections in endemic areas, and both are capable of infecting ticks.[9,10,17,24] Identification of dogs infected with *E ewingii* and/or *E chaffeensis* outside the range of *A americanum* (eg, Cameroon, Brazil, South Korea)[25–28] suggests other ticks, such as *R sanguineus*, may transmit these pathogens,[21] although a comprehensive documentation of multiple tick-borne disease agents in

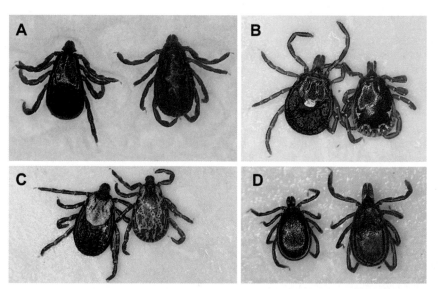

Fig. 1. Tick vectors of ehrlichiosis and anaplasmosis. (*A*) *Rhipicephalus sanguineus*, the brown dog tick. (*B*) *Amblyomma americanum*, the lone star tick. (*C*) *Dermacentor variabilis*, the American dog tick. (*D*) *Ixodes scapularis*, the eastern black-legged tick. (*Courtesy of Susan E. Little.*)

a heavily *R sanguineus* infested population of dogs did not reveal the presence of *E ewingii* or *E chaffeensis*.[29] Infection with *Ehrlichia* spp can also occur following blood subinoculation. The organisms survive and remain infectious in preserved, refrigerated whole blood, suggesting both exposure to contaminated needles and blood transfusions are viable, albeit uncommon, routes of infection.[30,31]

The ticks that vector *Ehrlichia* spp (*R sanguineus*, *A americanum*, *D variabilis*) are more active in the spring and summer months.[32] Dogs are more likely to become infected during these times,[10] and cases of ehrlichiosis are more common during warmer times of the year.[33] However, dogs with ehrlichiosis can present any month of the year. *R sanguineus*, which can survive indoors in homes or kennels, can be active at any time of the year and is particularly common year-round in subtropical areas such as the coastal southern United States.[32,34] In addition, clinical disease may not develop until a dog has been infected for several months or years and the ticks that transmitted the infection have long since detached. Neither time of year nor absence of ticks at presentation should eliminate the suspicion of canine ehrlichiosis in an individual patient.

Infection and Clinical Disease

The variety of *Ehrlichia* spp that infect dogs, together with documented variations in pathogenicity of different strains of *E canis*, results in a wide spectrum of disease ranging from clinically inapparent to severe, and which is further compounded by variations in individual dog and/or breed-specific immune responses, differences in the dose of pathogen transmitted during tick feeding, presence of coinfecting agents, and the overall health of the dog prior to infection.[33] In areas where vector tick populations are high and active throughout much of the year, a fairly high percentage of dogs may have antibodies to *Ehrlichia* spp. A summary report on testing dogs from throughout the United States identified counties in the South in which as many as 15% of the dogs tested had antibodies to *Ehrlichia* spp.[35] In another study focusing on dogs in a high-prevalence area in the south-central United States, 59% of dogs tested in one veterinary practice had antibodies to *E ewingii* and 25% had antibodies to *E chaffeensis*.[10] Because the commonly used patient-side assays for *E canis* will also pick up antibodies against some strains of *E chaffeensis*,[36] a relatively milder pathogen in dogs, and because strains of *E canis* vary in pathogenicity, many seropositive dogs may not have evidence of clinical disease. However, when clinical disease develops, both severe morbidity and mortality can occur.

Dogs with ehrlichiosis due to *E canis* infection may develop an acute or chronic febrile illness characterized by lethargy, anorexia, myalgia, splenomegaly, lymphadenopathy, and bleeding diatheses.[3,37] Acute disease usually develops within 2 to 4 weeks following tick transmission; disease may be more severe with certain strains of *E canis* and appears to be exacerbated when coinfections with other tick-borne rickettsial or protozoal pathogens occur.[38,39] Despite the severe nature of some cases of acute *E canis* infection, including fatalities, many dogs appear to tolerate infection without developing overt clinical disease. These dogs may enter a subclinical phase of infection in which they remain chronically infected for months to years but without overt evidence of disease; such dogs often have mild thrombocytopenia but no other evidence of pathology.[40]

For some dogs, however, a severe, potentially fatal form of chronic ehrlichiosis can develop months to years after initial infection with *E canis* in which fever, anorexia, and weight loss are accompanied by myalgia, bleeding tendencies, ocular lesions, and neurologic abnormalities.[3,37] Epistaxis (**Fig. 2**), petechial or ecchymotic hemorrhage, hyphema, retinal hemorrhage, and hematuria may develop; anterior uveitis with retinal

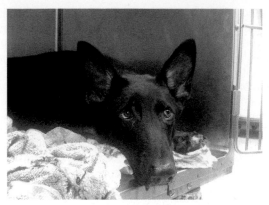

Fig. 2. Dog with severe epistaxis due to *Ehrlichia canis* infection. (*Courtesy of* Susan E. Little.)

changes is also described. Ataxia, head tilt, nystagmus, and seizures have been reported but are present in a minority of dogs with clinical ehrlichiosis.[33] Lameness may be observed in dogs infected with *E canis* alone but is thought to be caused by a reluctance to move due to myalgia rather than arthralgia. Although German Shepherd dogs appear to be particularly susceptible to developing disease caused by *E canis* infection,[41] severe disease may be seen in any dog that becomes infected with a moderately or highly pathogenic strain.[38]

Dogs with clinical disease due to *E ewingii* most commonly present with fever and lameness associated with a neutrophilic polyarthritis; neurologic signs, including ataxia, head tilt, and paresis are also reported.[42] Experimental infection with *E ewingii* also results in fever and thrombocytopenia.[7] In contrast, experimental infection with *E chaffeensis* alone generally produces mild disease,[4,43] although dogs that present clinically may be more severely affected,[5,44] perhaps due to the presence of coinfecting pathogens. Infection with *E chaffeensis*, like *E canis*, appears to persist in dogs[43] and thus the opportunity exists for development of disease as other pathogens are acquired over time. Uveitis and meningitis were present in dogs experimentally infected with *E canis* but were not identified in dogs with *E chaffeensis* or *E ewingii*.[45]

Clinical pathologic changes in dogs with ehrlichiosis include thrombocytopenia, pancytopenia, large granular lymphocytosis, hyperglobulinemia, hypoalbuminemia, and increased serum alanine aminotransferase; bone marrow hypoplasia can also occur with infection.[33,37] Decreased platelet function contributes to the bleeding diatheses seen in dogs with acute and chronic ehrlichiosis.[46] Decreased production of platelets from hypoplastic bone marrow, together with sequestration, increased consumption, and secretion of platelet-migration inhibition factor by lymphocytes exposed to *Ehrlichia*-infected cells, all contribute to both thrombocytopenia and clinical bleeding.[33,47] Although a polyclonal or monoclonal gammopathy may develop, high antibody titers do not protect against future infection or eliminate existing infections.[48] Rather, some of the pathology seen in ehrlichiosis appears to be immune complex mediated, and dogs with monoclonal gammopathy may develop sequelae such as glomerulopathy or subretinal hemorrhage.[33,49,50]

CANINE ANAPLASMOSIS
Agents of Canine Anaplasmosis

Dogs may be infected with both *Anaplasma phagocytophilum* and *Anaplasma platys*. The first reports of *A phagocytophilum* in dogs were from California in the early

1980s.[51] The organism was recognized as very similar to *Ehrlichia equi* in horses, and later, as closely resembling what was then referred to as the human granulocytic ehrlichiosis (HGE) agent first described from people in Minnesota and Wisconsin.[52,53] Analysis of phylogenetic relationships among *Ehrlichia* spp, *Anaplasma* spp, and *Neorickettsia* spp resulted in reclassification of these agents in 2001, synonymization of *E equi*, *E phagocytophila*, and the HGE agent, and movement of this organism into the genus *Anaplasma* as *A phagocytophilum*.[54]

The original strains comprising the genogroup *A phagocytophilum* remain distinct both in terms of species in which they cause disease and geographic distribution.[55] For example, isolates of *A phagocytophilum* from Europe did not cause disease when inoculated into horses, and isolates from humans in the United States failed to cause disease in cattle.[56] In addition, genetic variants of *A phagocytophilum* not associated with disease have been described.[57] Both infection and disease due to *A phagocytophilum* (HGE strain) is well recognized in dogs in areas of North America and Europe with dense populations of *Ixodes* spp ticks.[52,58–60]

A platys was first described from dogs in the United States in 1978 and has since been recognized worldwide.[61,62] Although not conclusively demonstrated, transmission is thought to occur via *R sanguineus* ticks, and *A platys* is more often identified from areas where *E canis*, another *R sanguineus* transmitted pathogen, is common, such as the southern United States.[10,35,61] Infection is also reported from dogs used in biomedical research.[63] Disease caused by *A platys* infection alone is relatively mild, but coinfection with other disease agents, including *E canis*, results in more severe clinical pathology.[61,64]

Tick Vectors, Reservoir Hosts, and Routes of Transmission

Ixodes spp ticks of the *Ixodes persulcatus* complex are the only recognized vectors of *A phagocytophilum*, with *Ixodes scapularis*, *Ixodes pacificus*, and *Ixodes ricinus* considered the predominant vectors in eastern North America, along the west coast of the United States, and in Europe, respectively.[65] A diverse array of vertebrates is susceptible to and is found to harbor infection with *A phagocytophilum* in nature; various rodent species, deer species, and birds are all considered potential reservoir hosts.[65,66] In areas of North America where disease due to *A phagocytophilum* commonly occurs in people and dogs, such as the northeastern and upper Midwestern United States and the West Coast, immature *Ixodes* spp vectors feed on rodents, and thus rodents are considered an important reservoir host in nature.[67–69] Infection with *A phagocytophilum* (HGE strain) has been identified in deer,[70,71] but the organisms appear to be variants (eg, *Ap*-VI, which does not infect mice[72]) that have not been reported as disease agents in dogs or people.[57,73] Although white-tailed deer are experimentally susceptible to infection with disease-associated variants,[74] transmission from deer to *I scapularis* ticks has only been demonstrated with the *Ap*-VI strain and not a human isolate,[75] and deer are not considered a reservoir host for disease-causing strains of *A phagocytophilum* in North America.[76]

The predominant tick vector of *A platys* is suspected to be *R sanguineus*.[61] Successful experimental work to confirm this cycle has not been reported to date,[77] but *A platys* has been repeatedly identified in *R sanguineus* ticks via polymerase chain reaction (PCR) assay as well as in *Dermacentor auratus* ticks in Thailand, and infection with *A platys* is common in dogs in areas with high *R sanguineus* pressure, such as the Caribbean.[29,78–82] Dogs, a strongly preferred host for *R sanguineus*, are considered the main reservoir host of *A platys*.[61,83,84] Infections with *A platys* in species other than dogs have not been confirmed to date. A cat was described with suspected *A platys* infection based on platelet inclusions, but experimental attempts to infect cats via blood subinoculation were not successful.[61,85] Electron microscopy and serology failed to confirm suspected cases of human infection with A platys in Venezuela.[86]

Anaplasma spp can also be transmitted directly via blood subinoculation, a route commonly used in experimental work, and by blood transfusion. A case of suspected human infection with A phagocytophilum following exposure to deer blood while cleaning carcasses was reported, although the source of infection could not be definitively ascertained.[87] Transfusion with blood products infected with A phagocytophilum was confirmed to be responsible for a human case in Minnesota,[88,89] and thus risk of infection on exposure to infected blood or contaminated needles exists. Nosocomial infection also has been reported in people and warrants further investigation.[90,91] Perinatal and transplacental transmission have also been confirmed in people and cattle, respectively, but not in dogs.[92–94]

Clinical Disease

Dogs with anaplasmosis due to A phagocytophilum infection almost invariably present with lethargy and fever, and most are anorexic. Lameness and reluctance to move due to development of a neutrophilic polyarthritis is also described; other clinical signs include vomiting, diarrhea, and bleeding diatheses such as epistaxis.[52,58–60] Following experimental inoculation with A phagocytophilum, dogs develop fever and depression.[95] Nonetheless, many if not most dogs remain apparently healthy following infection; in some areas where disease is endemic, as many as 60% of dogs may be serologically positive and the majority of these do not have overt evidence of clinical disease.[35,96] Canine infection with A phagocytophilum has historically been considered self-limiting, but recrudescence of infection on administration of prednisone several months after apparent resolution both with and without doxycycline treatment has been reported.[97,98]

Pathologic changes in dogs with disease due to A phagocytophilum resemble those seen in ehrlichiosis. Both splenomegaly and lymphadenopathy are reported and are thought to be associated with reactive lymphoid hyperplasia.[52,60] The great majority (>90%) of dogs with anaplasmosis due to A phagocytophilum develop thrombocytopenia,[52,58,60] presumably because of platelet destruction, as megakaryocytes are increased in bone marrow.[99] Additional changes reported include lymphopenia, mild anemia, which may be nonregenerative or regenerative, hyperglobulinemia, hypoalbuminemia, and increased alkaline phosphatase.[52,58,60]

Anaplasmosis caused by A platys induces a recurrent thrombocytopenia, which waxes and wanes on approximately a 10- to 14-day cycle during acute infection[62]; in the absence of other infecting agents or complicating factors, the thrombocytopenia can resolve without treatment, presumably due to development of an immune response, and most dogs infected with A platys in the United States do not develop clinical disease despite low platelet counts.[63] However, disease has been reported, including bleeding tendencies and bilateral anterior uveitis.[61,62,83,100] Geographic variations in strains of A platys may account, in part, for the differences in reported pathogenicity; A platys infections in Spain and Chile appear to be more pathogenic than those seen in North America.[62,63,83,101]

Disease in dogs infected with A platys appears to be more common when dogs are also infected with other tick-transmitted pathogens, such as E canis,[44,102,103] although this association is not always supported in natural infections.[104] Experimental work has shown that coinfection with A platys and E canis results in more severe anemia and thrombocytopenia than infection with either pathogen alone.[64] In addition to thrombocytopenia, dogs with A platys infection may develop nonregenerative anemia, leukopenia, hypoalbuminemia, hypocalcemia, and hypergammaglobulinemia.[105,106] Inhibition of platelet aggregation may contribute to the bleeding diatheses when they occur.[107]

FELINE EHRLICHIOSIS AND ANAPLASMOSIS
Agents of Feline Ehrlichiosis and Anaplasmosis

Although described, disease due to *Ehrlichia* spp and *Anaplasma* spp in cats is not well understood and appears rare compared with that in dogs.[108] Cats are susceptible to experimental infection with *A phagocytophilum*[109]; experimental trials with *E canis* have not been reported in cats. Naturally occurring infection and/or disease due to *Ehrlichia* spp and *Anaplasma* spp has been documented in cats, with the most common clinical presentation described as fever, lethargy, and anorexia.[110–116] Specific identification of a causative agent is not always achieved, but both *E canis*-like organisms and *A phagocytophilum* have been implicated in several cases through microscopy and/or PCR.[110–113,115,116]

Survey of feline blood samples has shown that 4.3% of cats in the United States and 30% of cats in endemic regions harbor antibodies reactive to *A phagocytophilum* on indirect fluorescent antibody (IFA) assay.[117,118] Serologic evidence of *Ehrlichia* spp was not identified in a survey of cats in North America,[119] but has been as high as 17.2% in cats in Spain.[120–122] Discordant serologic results in naturally infected, PCR-positive cats suggest that the utility of serologic assays for *Ehrlichia* spp in cats may be limited.[111,123] Although infections have been identified in individual sick cats, surveys using PCR have failed to generate molecular evidence of infection with either *Ehrlichia* spp or *Anaplasma* spp in healthy cats to date.[117,121,122,124–126]

Tick Vectors and Reservoir Hosts

Cats are not known to serve as a reservoir host for any *Ehrlichia* spp or *Anaplasma* spp. The pathogens are maintained in natural cycles as described earlier, and cats apparently become infected with these organisms when fed on by infected ticks. *R sanguineus*, the most common vector of *E canis* in dogs, rarely feeds on cats.[32] However, cats residing in homes with established populations of *R sanguineus* may be at higher risk of infection, and *E canis* can be transmitted by *D variabilis*, adults of which readily feed on cats.[15,32] Adult *A americanum* also are commonly found on cats[32] but reports of molecular evidence of infection with *E chaffeensis* or *E ewingii* in cats are lacking. *I scapularis* readily feeds on cats as both a nymph and adult,[32] and *Ixodes* spp ticks have been reported from cats with anaplasmosis due to *A phagocytophilum* infection at the time of presentation.[115,116]

Clinical Disease

Predominant signs reported in cats with ehrlichiosis include fever, anorexia, lethargy, myalgia, dyspnea, and enlarged lymph nodes.[108] Polyarthritis has also been reported[111] and anemia, thrombocytopenia, and pancytopenia are described.[108,111] Similar signs have been attributed to feline infection with *A phagocytophilum*, including fever, joint pain, lameness, enlarged lymph nodes, and weight loss, as well as periodontal disease, conjunctivitis, and neurologic signs.[112,115,116] Presence of infection has been confirmed by visualization of morulae on microscopy and/or PCR detection,[110–113,115,116] but culture isolation of an *Ehrlichia* sp or an *Anaplasma* sp from a cat has not yet been reported.

DIAGNOSIS OF EHRLICHIOSIS AND ANAPLASMOSIS

Diagnosis of ehrlichiosis or anaplasmosis usually begins with clinical evaluation of a febrile, myalgic patient. A history of tick exposure and complete blood work revealing thrombocytopenia and other characteristic abnormalities further raise the index of suspicion. Laboratory confirmation of a diagnosis can be achieved by serology or PCR, although other methods, such as examination of stained blood smears for morulae, may be rewarding for some agents during acute infection. To maximize the likelihood of reaching a diagnosis, both PCR and serologic assays should be performed together with careful examination of stained blood smears in any patient in which ehrlichiosis or anaplasmosis is suspected. Cell culture is generally reserved for specialized research laboratories and, of the agents discussed here, to date has only been achieved for *E canis*, *E chaffeensis*, and *A phagocytophilum*.

Direct Examination of Blood Smears

Identification of morulae within infected cells on stained blood smears allows direct, immediate confirmation of a diagnosis of ehrlichiosis or anaplasmosis (**Fig. 3**). Unfortunately, morulae are not present in large number in many infected animals, particularly those infected with the monocytotropic *E canis* or *E chaffeensis*, even in the presence of severe clinical disease.[3,127] Examination of a larger number of cells in buffy coat smears or preparations from bone marrow aspirates can increase the likelihood of identifying morulae of these agents, but chronically infected dogs are rarely rickettsemic to a level detectable microscopically.[3,4] In contrast, both *E ewingii* and *A phagocytophilum* may be found in granulocytes of acutely infected individuals.[128,129] Although morphologically indistinguishable from one another, once infected neutrophils are recognized the geographic origin and knowledge about the tick populations active in a given area can suggest the agent most likely responsible for disease. Morulae of *A platys* can be found within platelets[106] but, in some cases, may be difficult to distinguish reliably from platelet granules.

Polymerase Chain Reaction

If patients are rickettsemic at the time of sample collection, identification of infection with *Ehrlichia* spp or *Anaplasma* spp can readily be achieved through PCR-based assays at reference laboratories. A confirmed positive PCR result on a validated assay is considered evidence of infection, although techniques used vary among different diagnostic laboratories. External validation is a key component of any diagnostic platform; sensitivity may not always translate from plasmid controls to clinical samples, and unexpected cross-amplifications can occur. For example, 16S rDNA-based primers designed for *Ehrlichia* spp and *Anaplasma* spp may also amplify DNA of *Wolbachia* spp, resulting in positive results in microfilaremic dogs that would not be

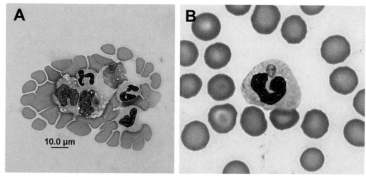

Fig. 3. Morulae of *Ehrlichia* spp. (*A*) *Ehrlichia canis* in a monocyte. (*B*) *Ehrlichia ewingii* in a neutrophil (note that *Anaplasma phagocytophilum* is morphologically identical to *E ewingii* on blood smear). (*Courtesy of* Robin W. Allison, Oklahoma State University, Stillwater, OK.)

identified without sequence confirmation.[130] Nonetheless, PCR assays have greatly enhanced our ability to identify infections with *Ehrlichia* sp and *Anaplasma* sp.

Negative results from a PCR test are more difficult to interpret and should not be used to rule out the presence of infection. Negative results may occur when organisms in circulation are below the level of detection, as may happen when infections progress or after initiation of antibiotic treatment, or because extraction has failed to remove PCR inhibitors in the sample. Blood samples to be submitted for PCR for *Ehrlichia* spp or *Anaplasma* spp ideally should be collected before administration of antibiotics and submitted to diagnostic laboratories with stringent quality control. In many diagnostic laboratories, PCR assays are available as panels for multiple agents. This approach enhances diagnostics, as coinfecting agents that may be present but not initially suspected can be identified and appropriately treated; in the absence of a comprehensive diagnostic panel, the presence of a coinfection may not be recognized until after the dog fails to respond to initial treatment attempts.

Serology

Long a mainstay of diagnosing ehrlichiosis or anaplasmosis, serologic assays remain useful for evaluating patients for evidence of infection with these agents. IFA assays for *E canis* and *A phagocytophilum* are widely available through diagnostic laboratories; cross-reactions among species within these genera and, to some extent, between the 2 genera, commonly occur, although infection with a related agent may generate a lower antibody titer than that with the primary agent.[8,131,132] Point-of-care assays developed to detect antibodies to specific peptides of *E canis* and *A phagocytophilum* (ie, 3Dx/4Dx SNAP, IDEXX Laboratories, Westbrook, ME, USA) are also commonly used. The *E canis* analyte on the 3Dx/4Dx SNAP assay will detect antibodies generated against some strains of *E chaffeensis*; the *A phagocytophilum* analyte will also react with antibodies generated against *A platys*.[36,133] Although developed for use in dogs, these assays are not species specific; the tests may be used for identifying antibodies to *Ehrlichia* spp, *Anaplasma* spp, and *Borrelia burgdorferi* in other species, including cats and horses.[134,135]

Regardless of the assay used, clinical disease can develop prior to seroconversion. Accordingly, a negative antibody test should not be used to eliminate a diagnosis of ehrlichiosis or anaplasmosis in an acutely ill patient.[136] Conversely, healthy dogs may have detectable antibodies without any apparent adverse effects, particularly when infected with *E chaffeensis*, which appears to be a relatively mild canine pathogen[4]; in one study, the majority of dogs with antibodies reactive to *E canis* on 3Dx/4Dx SNAP assay actually had exposure to *E chaffeensis* rather than *E canis*.[10] In addition, some dogs tolerate infection without developing overt clinical illness, and antibody titers may persist for months to years even after treatment and resolution of clinical signs.[137,138] Long-standing presence of antibodies is particularly common in dogs with *E canis*, presumably due to persistent infection or reinfection.[132] Because many dogs with antibodies to *Ehrlichia* spp or *Anaplasma* spp are clinically normal, the value of screening dogs for exposure to these organisms is not clear. In a study that evaluated the link between presence of antibodies and subclinical disease, 39% of dogs seropositive for *E canis* on a patient-side enzyme-linked immunosorbent assay were found to be thrombocytopenic,[139] suggesting these assays may allow identification of dogs with clinically inapparent, but nonetheless pathogenic, infections.

Dogs exposed to ticks can acquire additional infections over time; identifying and treating these infections early in the process could forestall or even prevent development of clinical disease. The current American College of Veterinary Internal Medicine

(AVCIM) consensus statement does not make a specific recommendation for or against routine screening.[140] Advantages of screening include the ability to identify and treat infected dogs, reducing both development of chronic disease and reservoir status within a kennel or population. Disadvantages of testing healthy dogs for antibodies to these agents are that positive dogs may be unnecessarily treated; treatment may not prevent development of chronic infection in some dogs, and, as with any antibiotic, treatment can have adverse effects.[140] When antibodies to *Ehrlichia* spp or *Anaplasma* spp are identified in an apparently healthy dog, blood tests including a complete blood count with a platelet count should be performed to evaluate for the presence of subclinical disease that may indicate treatment is needed.

TREATMENT AND PREVENTION OF EHRLICHIOSIS AND ANAPLASMOSIS

Doxycycline is considered the treatment of choice for both ehrlichiosis and anaplasmosis in dogs[55,140]; this antibiotic has also been used successfully in cats infected with these agents.[111,116] For ehrlichiosis, the AVCIM consensus statement recommends that doxycycline be administered at a dose of 10 mg/kg by mouth every 24 hours for 28 days.[140] Concerns regarding tooth discoloration with doxycycline are not supported by current literature and should not preclude the use of this antibiotic.[136] Although some studies report antibiotic clearance of ehrlichial infections, others have documented persistent infections after treatment with doxycycline using xenodiagnostic strategies, PCR on splenic aspirates, and culture isolation from treated dogs.[141–146] The reasons for these discordant results are not clear but differences in outcome may relate to route of initial infection (ie, tick feeding vs intravenous inoculation of organisms from cell culture), duration of infection prior to treatment, or duration of treatment itself.[143–145]

When treatment failure or recrudescence of disease occurs, additional administration of antimicrobials should be considered together with evaluation for concurrent disease. Although less commonly used, imidocarb is effective against *E canis*.[147,148] Imidocarb has the advantage of persistent activity following intramuscular administration; premedication with atropine can lessen the severity of adverse events associated with its use.[123] Fluoroquinolones, including enrofloxacin, are not effective against *Ehrlichia* spp but may have efficacy against *A phagocytophilum*.[149,150] Rifampin has been used successfully in people to treat *A phagocytophilum* infections[151,152] and also has been shown to be effective against *E canis* in dogs.[153] Penicillin and other β-lactam antibiotics are not effective against these agents.[140] The duration of treatment necessary to clear *A phagocytophilum* has not been completely evaluated; 14 days of doxycycline is commonly recommended[55] but concerns about persistent infections both with and without antibiotic treatment[97,98] lead many veterinarians to prescribe a longer (4-week) course similar to that used in treating ehrlichiosis and Lyme borreliosis.[140,154]

In most dogs with mild to moderate acute ehrlichiosis or anaplasmosis, clinical improvement is noted within 1 to 2 days of instituting antibiotic therapy.[55,123,140] However, dogs that present with more severe clinical disease or with chronic ehrlichiosis may take longer to respond.[55,123] In these cases, adjunctive therapy with a short course (7 days or less) of prednisone can be used to support clinical improvement early in treatment by addressing the inflammation directly.[33,123] This approach also has clinical utility early in treatment when laboratory confirmation of ehrlichiosis is pending, and immune-mediated thrombocytopenia remains a potential clinical diagnosis.[33,123] Other supportive treatments, including blood transfusion, parenteral fluid administration, and/or management of glomerulonephritis, may be indicated in individual cases and have been discussed previously.[123,140,155]

Dogs remain susceptible to reinfection with *E canis* and *E chaffeensis* following successful resolution of primary infection, although disease induced by reinfection with a homologous strain was less severe,[5,141] suggesting some protective immunity may develop. One study found a horse was resistant to reinfection with *A phagocytophilum*.[156] A case report documents that *A phagocytophilum* reinfection can occur in people, although it appears to be rare.[157] When reinfection and subsequent clinical disease occurs, additional courses of treatment are indicated. Vaccines are not available to prevent infection with these organisms in dogs or people. Prophylactic administration of tetracycline antibiotics has been used to prevent canine ehrlichiosis during outbreaks[158] but is considered impractical and potentially problematic. Stringent attention to tick control is the only available means of preventing infection with *Ehrlichia* sp or *Anaplasma* sp.

Routine, consistent (monthly) application of topical acaricides, including imidacloprid/permethrin and fipronil, have been shown to prevent infection with these organisms, as evidenced by decreased seroconversion in protected dogs in experimental and natural transmission studies.[159–161] Routine, year-round use of acaricides on dogs is recommended because different stages and species of ticks are active throughout the year in many areas, onset of tick activity is somewhat unpredictable, and pets may travel. However, no acaricide is entirely effective at eliminating all ticks, and infection and disease has been reported in dogs receiving acaricides.[60] Prompt removal of attached ticks using forceps or gloved fingers is recommended to prevent infection. Additional strategies to reduce tick infestations include restricting access to tick-infested areas, managing the habitat around the home to discourage ticks, and selective, judicious use of acaricides in the environment.[136]

ZOONOTIC IMPLICATIONS OF EHRLICHIOSIS AND ANAPLASMOSIS IN DOGS AND CATS

With the exception of *A platys*, the *Ehrlichia* spp and *Anaplasma* spp that cause disease in pets are known to be zoonotic disease agents.[136] *E chaffeensis* and *A phagocytophilum* are well-known human pathogens, inducing HME and human anaplasmosis (formerly known as human granulocytotropic ehrlichiosis, or HGE), respectively[162,163]; *E ewingii* and *E canis* may also occasionally infect people.[8,164] Disease in people presents as a febrile, flu-like illness with myalgia, headache, and disorientation predominant clinical signs. Human monocytic ehrlichiosis is the most severe, with hospitalizations common and a fatality rate of up to 3%.[162] As with pets, infection is transmitted to people via tick feeding, and pets are not thought to increase the risk of these infections in people. However, blood subinoculation will result in transmission of infection, and thus care must be taken when handling blood or tissues from potentially infected animals, including dogs and cats. Recommendations for preventing infection in people are similar to those for pets, with a focus on tick control, and should include efforts to control ticks on pets and in the environment.[136]

REFERENCES

1. Donatien A, Lestoquard F. State of the present knowledge concerning rickettsiosis of animals. Arch Inst Pasteur Alger 1937;15:142–87.
2. Ewing SA. Observations on leukocytic inclusion bodies from dogs infected with *Babesia canis*. J Am Vet Med Assoc 1963;143:503–6.
3. Harrus S, Waner T. Diagnosis of canine monocytotropic ehrlichiosis (*Ehrlichia canis*): an overview. Vet J, in press. DOI:10.1016/j.tvjl.2010.02.001.

4. Dawson JE, Ewing SA. Susceptibility of dogs to infection with *Ehrlichia chaffeen-sis*, causative agent of human ehrlichiosis. Am J Vet Res 1992;53(8):1322–7.

5. Breitschwerdt EB, Hegarty BC, Hancock SI. Sequential evaluation of dogs natu-rally infected with *Ehrlichia canis*, *Ehrlichia chaffeensis*, *Ehrlichia equi*, *Ehrlichia ewingii*, or *Bartonella vinsonii*. J Clin Microbiol 1998;36(9):2645–51.

6. Ewing SA, Roberson WR, Buckner RG, et al. A new strain of *Ehrlichia canis*. J Am Vet Med Assoc 1971;159(12):1771–4.

7. Anziani OS, Ewing SA, Barker RW. Experimental transmission of a granulocytic form of the tribe Ehrlichieae by *Dermacentor variabilis* and *Amblyomma ameri-canum* to dogs. Am J Vet Res 1990;51(6):929–31.

8. Buller RS, Arens M, Hmiel SP, et al. *Ehrlichia ewingii*, a newly recognized agent of human ehrlichiosis. N Engl J Med 1999;341(3):148–55.

9. Liddell AM, Stockham SL, Scott MA, et al. Predominance of *Ehrlichia ewingii* in Missouri dogs. J Clin Microbiol 2003;41(10):4617–22.

10. Little SE, O'Connor TP, Hempstead J, et al. *Ehrlichia ewingii* infection and expo-sure rates in dogs from the southcentral United States. Vet Parasitol, in press. DOI:10.1016/j.vetpar.2010.05.006.

11. Groves MG, Dennis GL, Amyx HL, et al. Transmission of *Ehrlichia canis* to dogs by ticks (*Rhipicephalus sanguineus*). Am J Vet Res 1975;36(7):937–40.

12. Bremer WG, Schaefer JJ, Wagner ER, et al. Transstadial and intrastadial exper-imental transmission of *Ehrlichia canis* by male *Rhipicephalus sanguineus*. Vet Parasitol 2005;131(1–2):95–105.

13. Little SE, Hostetler J, Kocan KM. Movement of *Rhipicephalus sanguineus* adults between co-housed dogs during active feeding. Vet Parasitol 2007;150(1–2): 139–45.

14. Dantas-Torres F. The brown dog tick, *Rhipicephalus sanguineus* (Latreille, 1806) (Acari: Ixodidae): from taxonomy to control. Vet Parasitol 2008; 152(3–4):173–85.

15. Johnson EM, Ewing SA, Barker RW, et al. Experimental transmission of *Ehrlichia canis* (Rickettsiales: Ehrlichieae) by *Dermacentor variabilis* (Acari: Ixodidae). Vet Parasitol 1998;74(2–4):277–88.

16. Yabsley MJ. Natural history of *Ehrlichia chaffeensis*: vertebrate hosts and tick vectors from the United States and evidence for endemic transmission in other countries. Vet Parasitol 2010;167(2–4):136–48.

17. Murphy GL, Ewing SA, Whitworth LC, et al. A molecular and serologic survey of *Ehrlichia canis*, *E. chaffeensis*, and *E. ewingii* in dogs and ticks from Oklahoma. Vet Parasitol 1998;79(4):325–39.

18. Kocan AA, Levesque GC, Whitworth LC, et al. Naturally occurring *Ehrlichia chaffeensis* infection in coyotes from Oklahoma. Emerg Infect Dis 2000; 6(5):477–80.

19. Roland WE, Everett ED, Cyr TL, et al. *Ehrlichia chaffeensis* in Missouri ticks. Am J Trop Med Hyg 1998;59(4):641–3.

20. Gutierrez CN, Martinez M, Sanchez E, et al. Cultivation and molecular identifica-tion of *Ehrlichia canis* and *Ehrlichia chaffeensis* from a naturally co-infected dog in Venezuela. Vet Clin Pathol 2008;37(3):258–65.

21. Ndip LM, Ndip RN, Esemu SN, et al. Predominance of *Ehrlichia chaffeensis* in *Rhipicephalus sanguineus* ticks from kennel-confined dogs in Limbe, Cameroon. Exp Appl Acarol 2010;50(2):163–8.

22. Childs JE, Paddock CD. The ascendancy of *Amblyomma americanum* as a vector of pathogens affecting humans in the United States. Annu Rev Entomol 2003;48:307–37.

23. Cohen SB, Yabsley MJ, Freye JD, et al. Prevalence of *Ehrlichia chaffeensis* and *Ehrlichia ewingii* in ticks from Tennessee. Vector Borne Zoonotic Dis 2010;10(5): 435–40.
24. Yabsley MJ, Varela AS, Tate CM, et al. *Ehrlichia ewingii* infection in white-tailed deer (*Odocoileus virginianus*). Emerg Infect Dis 2002;8(7):668–71.
25. Ndip LM, Ndip RN, Esemu SN, et al. ehrlichial infection in Cameroonian canines by *Ehrlichia canis* and *Ehrlichia ewingii*. Vet Microbiol 2005; 111(1–2):59–66.
26. Ndip LM, Ndip RN, Ndive VE, et al. *Ehrlichia* species in *Rhipicephalus sanguineus* ticks in Cameroon. Vector Borne Zoonotic Dis 2007;7(2):221–7.
27. Oliveira LS, Oliveira KA, Mourao LC, et al. First report of *Ehrlichia ewingii* detected by molecular investigation in dogs from Brazil. Clin Microbiol Infect 2009;15(Suppl 1):55–6.
28. Yu DH, Li YH, Yoon JS, et al. *Ehrlichia chaffeensis* infection in dogs in South Korea. Vector Borne Zoonotic Dis 2008;8(3):355–8.
29. Yabsley MJ, McKibben J, Macpherson CN, et al. Prevalence of *Ehrlichia canis*, *Anaplasma platys*, *Babesia canis vogeli*, *Hepatozoon canis*, *Bartonella vinsonii berkhoffii*, and *Rickettsia* spp. in dogs from Grenada. Vet Parasitol 2008; 151(2–4):279–85.
30. McKechnie DB, Slater KS, Childs JE, et al. Survival of *Ehrlichia chaffeensis* in refrigerated, ADSOL-treated RBCs. Transfusion 2000;40(9):1041–7.
31. McQuiston JH, Childs JE, Chamberland ME, et al. Transmission of tick-borne agents of disease by blood transfusion: a review of known and potential risks in the United States. Transfusion 2000;40(3):274–84.
32. Dryden MW, Payne PA. Biology and control of ticks infesting dogs and cats in North America. Vet Ther 2004;5(2):139–54.
33. Neer TM, Harrus S. Canine monocytotropic ehrlichiosis and neorickettsiosis (*E. canis*, *E. chaffeensis*, *E. ruminantium*, *N. sennetsu*, and *N. risticii* infections). In: Greene CE, editor. Infectious diseases of the dog and cat. 3rd edition. St Louis (MO): Saunders Elsevier; 2006. p. 203–16.
34. Dantas-Torres F. Biology and ecology of the brown dog tick, *Rhipicephalus sanguineus*. Parasit Vectors 2010;3:26.
35. Bowman D, Little SE, Lorentzen L, et al. Prevalence and geographic distribution of *Dirofilaria immitis*, *Borrelia burgdorferi*, *Ehrlichia canis*, and *Anaplasma phagocytophilum* in dogs in the United States: results of a national clinic-based serologic survey. Vet Parasitol 2009;160(1–2):138–48.
36. O'Connor TP, Hanscom JL, Hegarty BC, et al. Comparison of an indirect immunofluorescence assay, Western blot analysis, and a commercially available ELISA for detection of *Ehrlichia canis* antibodies in canine sera. Am J Vet Res 2006;67(2):206–10.
37. Stich RW, Schaefer JJ, Bremer WG, et al. Host surveys, ixodid tick biology and transmission scenarios as related to the tick-borne pathogen, *Ehrlichia canis*. Vet Parasitol 2008;158(4):256–73.
38. Unver A, Rikihisa Y, Karaman M, et al. An acute severe ehrlichiosis in a dog experimentally infected with a new virulent strain of *Ehrlichia canis*. Clin Microbiol Infect 2008;15(Suppl 1):1–3.
39. Gal A, Harrus S, Arcoh I, et al. Coinfection with multiple tick-borne and intestinal parasites in a 6-week-old dog. Can Vet J 2007;48(6):619–22.
40. Waner T, Harrus S, Bark H, et al. Characterization of the subclinical phase of canine ehrlichiosis in experimentally infected beagle dogs. Vet Parasitol 1997; 69(3–4):307–17.

41. Nyindo M, Huxsoll DL, Ristic M, et al. Cell-mediated and humoral immune responses of German Shepherd Dogs and Beagles to experimental infection with *Ehrlichia canis*. Am J Vet Res 1980;41(2):250–4.

42. Goodman RA, Hawkins EC, Olby NJ, et al. Molecular identification of *Ehrlichia ewingii* infection in dogs: 15 cases (1997-2001). J Am Vet Med Assoc 2003; 222(8):1102–7.

43. Zhang XF, Zhang JZ, Long SW, et al. Experimental *Ehrlichia chaffeensis* infection in beagles. J Med Microbiol 2003;52(Pt 11):1021–6.

44. Kordick SK, Breitschwerdt EB, Hegarty BC, et al. Coinfection with multiple tick-borne pathogens in a Walker Hound kennel in North Carolina. J Clin Microbiol 1999;37(8):2631–8.

45. Panciera RJ, Ewing SA, Confer AW. Ocular histopathology of ehrlichial infections in the dog. Vet Pathol 2001;38(1):43–6.

46. Harrus S, Waner T, Eldor A, et al. Platelet dysfunction associated with experimental acute canine ehrlichiosis. Vet Rec 1996;139(12):290–3.

47. Abeygunawardena I, Kakoma I, Smith RD. Pathophysiology of canine ehrlichiosis. In: Williams JC, Kakoma I, editors. Ehrlichiosis: a vector-borne disease of animals and humans. Dordrecht (Netherland): Kluwer; 1990. p. 78–92.

48. Ristic M, Holland CJ. Canine ehrlichiosis. In: Woldehiwet Z, Ristic M, editors. Rickettsial and chlamydial diseases of domestic animals. Oxford: Pergamon Press; 1993. p. 169–86.

49. Harrus S, Ofri R, Aizenberg I, et al. Acute blindness associated with monoclonal gammopathy induced by *Ehrlichia canis* infection. Vet Parasitol 1998;78(2):155–60.

50. Luckschander N, Kleiter M, Willmann M. [Renal amyloidosis caused by *Ehrlichia canis*]. Schweiz Arch Tierheilkd 2003;145(10):482–5 [in German].

51. Madewell BR, Gribble DH. Infection in two dogs with an agent resembling *Ehrlichia equi*. J Am Vet Med Assoc 1982;180(5):512–4.

52. Greig B, Asanovich KM, Armstrong PJ, et al. Geographic, clinical, serologic, and molecular evidence of granulocytic ehrlichiosis, a likely zoonotic disease, in Minnesota and Wisconsin dogs. J Clin Microbiol 1996;34(1):44–8.

53. Bakken JS, Dumler JS, Chen SM, et al. Human granulocytic ehrlichiosis in the upper Midwest United States. A new species emerging? JAMA 1994;272(3):212–8.

54. Dumler JS, Barbet AF, Bekker CP, et al. Reorganization of genera in the families Rickettsiaceae and Anaplasmataceae in the order Rickettsiales: unification of some species of *Ehrlichia* with *Anaplasma*, *Cowdria* with *Ehrlichia* and *Ehrlichia* with *Neorickettsia*, descriptions of six new species combinations and designation of *Ehrlichia equi* and 'HGE agent' as subjective synonyms of *Ehrlichia phagocytophila*. Int J Syst Evol Microbiol 2001;51(Pt 6):2145–65.

55. Carrade DD, Foley JE, Borjesson DL, et al. Canine granulocytic anaplasmosis: a review. J Vet Intern Med 2009;23(6):1129–41.

56. Pusterla N, Pusterla JB, Braun U, et al. Experimental cross-infections with *Ehrlichia phagocytophila* and human granulocytic ehrlichia-like agent in cows and horses. Vet Rec 1999;145(11):311–4.

57. Courtney JW, Dryden RL, Montgomery J, et al. Molecular characterization of *Anaplasma phagocytophilum* and *Borrelia burgdorferi* in *Ixodes scapularis* ticks from Pennsylvania. J Clin Microbiol 2003;41(4):1569–73.

58. Poitout FM, Shinozaki JK, Stockwell PJ, et al. Genetic variants of *Anaplasma phagocytophilum* infecting dogs in Western Washington State. J Clin Microbiol 2005;43(2):796–801.

59. Egenvall AE, Hedhammar AA, Bjoersdorff AI. Clinical features and serology of 14 dogs affected by granulocytic ehrlichiosis in Sweden. Vet Rec 1997;140(9):222–6.

60. Kohn B, Galke D, Beelitz P, et al. Clinical features of canine granulocytic anaplasmosis in 18 naturally infected dogs. J Vet Intern Med 2008;22(6): 1289–95.
61. Harvey JW. Thrombocytotropic anaplasmosis (*A. platys* infection). In: Greene CE, editor. Infectious diseases of the dog and cat. 3rd edition. St. Louis (MO): Saunders Elsevier; 2006. p. 229–31.
62. Harvey JW, Simpson CF, Gaskin JM. Cyclic thrombocytopenia induced by a *Rickettsia*-like agent in dogs. J Infect Dis 1978;137(2):182–8.
63. Bradfield JF, Vore SJ, Pryor WH Jr. *Ehrlichia platys* infection in dogs. Lab Anim Sci 1996;46(5):565–8.
64. Gaunt S, Beall M, Stillman B, et al. Experimental infection and co-infection of dogs with *Anaplasma platys* and *Ehrlichia canis*: hematologic, serologic and molecular findings. Parasit Vectors 2010;3(1):33.
65. Woldehiwet Z. The natural history of *Anaplasma phagocytophilum*. Vet Parasitol 2010;167(2–4):108–22.
66. Greig B, Armstrong PJ. Canine granulocytotropic anaplasmosis (*A. phagocytophilum* infection). In: Greene CE, editor. Infectious diseases of the dog and cat. St Louis (MO): Saunders Elsevier; 2006. p. 219–24.
67. Nicholson WL, Muir S, Sumner JW, et al. Serologic evidence of infection with *Ehrlichia* spp. in wild rodents (*Muridae*: Sigmodontinae) in the United States. J Clin Microbiol 1998;36(3):695–700.
68. Stafford KC 3rd, Massung RF, Magnarelli LA, et al. Infection with agents of human granulocytic ehrlichiosis, Lyme disease, and babesiosis in wild white-footed mice (*Peromyscus leucopus*) in Connecticut. J Clin Microbiol 1999; 37(9):2887–92.
69. DeNatale CE, Burkot TR, Schneider BS, et al. Novel potential reservoirs for *Borrelia* sp. and the agent of human granulocytic ehrlichiosis in Colorado. J Wildl Dis 2002;38(2):478–82.
70. Belongia EA, Reed KD, Mitchell PD, et al. Prevalence of granulocytic *Ehrlichia* infection among white-tailed deer in Wisconsin. J Clin Microbiol 1997;35(6): 1465–8.
71. Dugan VG, Yabsley MJ, Tate CM, et al. Evaluation of white-tailed deer (*Odocoileus virginianus*) as natural sentinels for *Anaplasma phagocytophilum*. Vector Borne Zoonotic Dis 2006;6(2):192–207.
72. Massung RF, Priestley RA, Miller NJ, et al. Inability of a variant strain of *Anaplasma phagocytophilum* to infect mice. J Infect Dis 2003;188(11):1757–63.
73. Morissette E, Massung RF, Foley JE, et al. Diversity of *Anaplasma phagocytophilum* strains, USA. Emerg Infect Dis 2009;15(6):928–31.
74. Tate CM, Mead DG, Luttrell MP, et al. Experimental infection of white-tailed deer with *Anaplasma phagocytophilum*, etiologic agent of human granulocytic anaplasmosis. J Clin Microbiol 2005;43(8):3595–601.
75. Reichard MV, Roman RM, Kocan KM, et al. Inoculation of white-tailed deer (*Odocoileus virginianus*) with Ap-V1 Or NY-18 strains of *Anaplasma phagocytophilum* and microscopic demonstration of Ap-V1 In *Ixodes scapularis* adults that acquired infection from deer as nymphs. Vector Borne Zoonotic Dis 2009;9(5): 565–8.
76. Massung RF, Courtney JW, Hiratzka SL, et al. *Anaplasma phagocytophilum* in white-tailed deer. Emerg Infect Dis 2005;11(10):1604–6.
77. Simpson RM, Gaunt SD, Hair JA, et al. Evaluation of *Rhipicephalus sanguineus* as a potential biologic vector of *Ehrlichia platys*. Am J Vet Res 1991;52(9): 1537–41.

78. Inokuma H, Raoult D, Brouqui P. Detection of *Ehrlichia platys* DNA in brown dog ticks (*Rhipicephalus sanguineus*) in Okinawa Island, Japan. J Clin Microbiol 2000;38(11):4219–21.

79. Motoi Y, Satoh H, Inokuma H, et al. First detection of *Ehrlichia platys* in dogs and ticks in Okinawa, Japan. Microbiol Immunol 2001;45(1):89–91.

80. Sanogo YO, Davoust B, Inokuma H, et al. First evidence of *Anaplasma platys* in *Rhipicephalus sanguineus* (Acari: Ixodida) collected from dogs in Africa. Onderstepoort J Vet Res 2003;70(3):205–12.

81. Sarih M, M'Ghirbi Y, Bouattour A, et al. Detection and identification of *Ehrlichia* spp. in ticks collected in Tunisia and Morocco. J Clin Microbiol 2005;43(3): 1127–32.

82. Parola P, Cornet JP, Sanogo YO, et al. Detection of *Ehrlichia* spp., *Anaplasma* spp., *Rickettsia* spp., and other eubacteria in ticks from the Thai-Myanmar border and Vietnam. J Clin Microbiol 2003;41(4):1600–8.

83. Abarca K, Lopez J, Perret C, et al. *Anaplasma platys* in dogs, Chile. Emerg Infect Dis 2007;13(9):1392–5.

84. Eddlestone SM, Gaunt SD, Neer TM, et al. PCR detection of *Anaplasma platys* in blood and tissue of dogs during acute phase of experimental infection. Exp Parasitol 2007;115(2):205–10.

85. Santarem VA, Laposy CB, Farias MR. *Ehrlichia platys*-like inclusions and morulae in platelets of a cat [abstract]. Brazilian J Vet Sci 2000;7:130.

86. Arraga-Alvarado C, Palmar M, Parra O, et al. Fine structural characterisation of a *Rickettsia*-like organism in human platelets from patients with symptoms of ehrlichiosis. J Med Microbiol 1999;48(11):991–7.

87. Bakken JS, Krueth JK, Lund T, et al. Exposure to deer blood may be a cause of human granulocytic ehrlichiosis. Clin Infect Dis 1996;23(1):198.

88. Centers for Disease Control and Prevention (CDC). *Anaplasma phagocytophilum* transmitted through blood transfusion—Minnesota, 2007. MMWR Morb Mortal Wkly Rep 2008;57(42):1145–8.

89. Waxman M. Update on emerging infections: news from the Centers for Disease Control and Prevention. *Anaplasma phagocytophilum* transmitted through blood transfusion—Minnesota 2007. Ann Emerg Med 2009;53(5):643–6.

90. Zhang L, Liu Y, Ni D, et al. Nosocomial transmission of human granulocytic anaplasmosis in China. JAMA 2008;300(19):2263–70.

91. Krause PJ, Wormser GP. Nosocomial transmission of human granulocytic anaplasmosis? JAMA 2008;300(19):2308–9.

92. Plier ML, Breitschwerdt EB, Hegarty BC, et al. Lack of evidence for perinatal transmission of canine granulocytic anaplasmosis from a bitch to her offspring. J Am Anim Hosp Assoc 2009;45(5):232–8.

93. Pusterla N, Braun U, Wolfensberger C, et al. Intrauterine infection with *Ehrlichia phagocytophila* in a cow. Vet Rec 1997;141(4):101–2.

94. Horowitz HW, Kilchevsky E, Haber S, et al. Perinatal transmission of the agent of human granulocytic ehrlichiosis. N Engl J Med 1998;339(6):375–8.

95. Egenvall A, Bjoersdorff A, Lilliehook I, et al. Early manifestations of granulocytic ehrlichiosis in dogs inoculated experimentally with a Swedish *Ehrlichia* species isolate. Vet Rec 1998;143(15):412–7.

96. Beall MJ, Chandrashekar R, Eberts MD, et al. Serological and molecular prevalence of Borrelia burgdorferi, *Anaplasma phagocytophilum*, and *Ehrlichia* species in dogs from Minnesota. Vector Borne Zoonotic Dis 2008;8(4):455–64.

97. Egenvall A, Lilliehook I, Bjoersdorff A, et al. Detection of granulocytic *Ehrlichia* species DNA by PCR in persistently infected dogs. Vet Rec 2000;146(7):186–90.

98. Alleman AR, Chandrashekar R, Beall M. Experimental inoculation of dogs with a human isolate (NY18) of *Anaplasma phagocytophilum* and demonstration of persistent infection following doxycycline therapy [abstract]. J Vet Intern Med 2006;20:763.

99. Lilliehook I, Egenvall A, Tvedten HW. Hematopathology in dogs experimentally infected with a Swedish granulocytic *Ehrlichia* species. Vet Clin Pathol 1998; 27(4):116–22.

100. Glaze MB, Gaunt SD. Uveitis associated with *Ehrlichia platys* infection in a dog. J Am Vet Med Assoc 1986;189(8):916–7.

101. Aguirre E, Tesouro MA, Ruiz L, et al. Genetic characterization of *Anaplasma* (*Ehrlichia*) *platys* in dogs in Spain. J Vet Med A Physiol Pathol Clin Med 2006; 53(4):197–200.

102. Hua P, Yuhai M, Shide T, et al. Canine ehrlichiosis caused simultaneously by *Ehrlichia canis* and *Ehrlichia platys*. Microbiol Immunol 2000;44(9):737–9.

103. Suksawat J, Pitulle C, Arraga-Alvarado C, et al. Coinfection with three *Ehrlichia* species in dogs from Thailand and Venezuela with emphasis on consideration of 16S ribosomal DNA secondary structure. J Clin Microbiol 2001;39(1):90–3.

104. Mylonakis ME, Koutinas AF, Breitschwerdt EB, et al. Chronic canine ehrlichiosis (*Ehrlichia canis*): a retrospective study of 19 natural cases. J Am Anim Hosp Assoc 2004;40(3):174–84.

105. Baker DC, Gaunt SD, Babin SS. Anemia of inflammation in dogs infected with *Ehrlichia platys*. Am J Vet Res 1988;49(7):1014–6.

106. Baker DC, Simpson M, Gaunt SD, et al. Acute *Ehrlichia platys* infection in the dog. Vet Pathol 1987;24(5):449–53.

107. Gaunt SD, Baker DC, Babin SS. Platelet aggregation studies in dogs with acute *Ehrlichia platys* infection. Am J Vet Res 1990;51(2):290–3.

108. Stubbs CJ, Holland CH, Relf JS. Feline ehrlichiosis. Compendium on Continuing Education for the Practicing Veterinarian 2000;22(4):307–18.

109. Lewis GE Jr, Huxsoll DL, Ristic M, et al. Experimentally induced infection of dogs, cats, and nonhuman primates with *Ehrlichia equi*, etiologic agent of equine ehrlichiosis. Am J Vet Res 1975;36(1):85–8.

110. Buoro IB, Atwell RB, Kiptoon JC, et al. Feline anaemia associated with *Ehrlichia*-like bodies in three domestic short-haired cats. Vet Rec 1989;125(17):434–6.

111. Breitschwerdt EB, Abrams-Ogg AC, Lappin MR, et al. Molecular evidence supporting *Ehrlichia canis*-like infection in cats. J Vet Intern Med 2002; 16(6):642–9.

112. Tarello W. Microscopic and clinical evidence for *Anaplasma* (*Ehrlichia*) phagocytophilum infection in Italian cats. Vet Rec 2005;156(24):772–4.

113. Bouloy RP, Lappin MR, Holland CH, et al. Clinical ehrlichiosis in a cat. J Am Vet Med Assoc 1994;204(9):1475–8.

114. Peavy GM, Holland CJ, Dutta SK, et al. Suspected ehrlichial infection in five cats from a household. J Am Vet Med Assoc 1997;210(2):231–4.

115. Bjoersdorff A, Svendenius L, Owens JH, et al. Feline granulocytic ehrlichiosis— a report of a new clinical entity and characterisation of the infectious agent. J Small Anim Pract 1999;40(1):20–4.

116. Lappin MR, Breitschwerdt EB, Jensen WA, et al. Molecular and serologic evidence of *Anaplasma phagocytophilum* infection in cats in North America. J Am Vet Med Assoc 2004;225(6):893–6, 79.

117. Billeter SA, Spencer JA, Griffin B, et al. Prevalence of *Anaplasma phagocytophilum* in domestic felines in the United States. Vet Parasitol 2007;147(1–2): 194–8.

118. Magnarelli LA, Bushmich SL, IJdo JW, et al. Seroprevalence of antibodies against *Borrelia burgdorferi* and *Anaplasma phagocytophilum* in cats. Am J Vet Res 2005;66(11):1895–9.

119. Hackett TB, Jensen WA, Lehman TL, et al. Prevalence of DNA of *Mycoplasma haemofelis*, 'Candidatus *Mycoplasma haemominutum*,' *Anaplasma phagocytophilum*, and species of *Bartonella*, *Neorickettsia*, and *Ehrlichia* in cats used as blood donors in the United States. J Am Vet Med Assoc 2006;229(5):700–5.

120. Ortuno A, Gauss CB, Garcia F, et al. Serological evidence of *Ehrlichia* spp. exposure in cats from northeastern Spain. J Vet Med A Physiol Pathol Clin Med 2005;52(5):246–8.

121. Aguirre E, Tesouro MA, Amusategui I, et al. Assessment of feline ehrlichiosis in central Spain using serology and a polymerase chain reaction technique. Ann N Y Acad Sci 2004;1026:103–5.

122. Solano-Gallego L, Hegarty B, Espada Y, et al. Serological and molecular evidence of exposure to arthropod-borne organisms in cats from northeastern Spain. Vet Microbiol 2006;118(3–4):274–7.

123. Cohn LA. Ehrlichiosis and related infections. Vet Clin North Am Small Anim Pract 2003;33(4):863–84.

124. Ishak AM, Radecki S, Lappin MR. Prevalence of *Mycoplasma haemofelis*, 'Candidatus *Mycoplasma haemominutum*', *Bartonella* species, *Ehrlichia* species, and *Anaplasma phagocytophilum* DNA in the blood of cats with anemia. J Feline Med Surg 2007;9(1):1–7.

125. Eberhardt JM, Neal K, Shackelford T, et al. Prevalence of selected infectious disease agents in cats from Arizona. J Feline Med Surg 2006;8(3):164–8.

126. Lappin MR, Griffin B, Brunt J, et al. Prevalence of *Bartonella* species, *Haemoplasma* species, *Ehrlichia* species, *Anaplasma phagocytophilum*, and *Neorickettsia risticii* DNA in the blood of cats and their fleas in the United States. J Feline Med Surg 2006;8(2):85–90.

127. Dawson JE, Ewing SA, Davidson WR, et al. Human monocytotropic ehrlichiosis. In: Goodman JL, Dennis DT, Sonenshine DE, editors. Tick-borne diseases of humans. Washington, DC: ASM Press; 2005. p. 239–57.

128. Paddock C, Liddell AM, Storch GA. Other causes of tick-borne ehrlichioses, including *Ehrlichia ewingii*. In: Goodman JL, Dennis DT, Sonenshine DE, editors. Tick-borne diseases of humans. Washington, DC: ASM Press; 2005. p. 258–67.

129. Goodman JL. Human granulocytic anaplasmosis (ehrlichiosis). In: Goodman JL, Dennis DT, Sonenshine DE, editors. Tick-borne diseases of humans. Washington, DC: ASM Press; 2005. p. 218–38.

130. Unver A, Rikihisa Y, Kawahara M, et al. Analysis of 16S rRNA gene sequences of *Ehrlichia canis*, *Anaplasma platys*, and *Wolbachia* species from canine blood in Japan. Ann N Y Acad Sci 2003;990:692–8.

131. Paddock CD, Folk SM, Shore GM, et al. Infections with *Ehrlichia chaffeensis* and *Ehrlichia ewingii* in persons coinfected with human immunodeficiency virus. Clin Infect Dis 2001;33(9):1586–94.

132. Waner T, Harrus S, Jongejan F, et al. Significance of serological testing for ehrlichial diseases in dogs with special emphasis on the diagnosis of canine monocytic ehrlichiosis caused by *Ehrlichia canis*. Vet Parasitol 2001;95(1):1–15.

133. Diniz PP, Beall MJ, Omark K, et al. High prevalence of tick-borne pathogens in dogs from an Indian reservation in northeastern Arizona. Vector Borne Zoonotic Dis 2010;10(2):117–23.

134. Levy SA, O'Connor TP, Hanscom JL, et al. Evaluation of a canine C6 ELISA Lyme disease test for the determination of the infection status of cats naturally exposed to *Borrelia burgdorferi*. Vet Ther 2003;4(2):172–7.

135. Johnson AL, Divers TJ, Chang YF. Validation of an in-clinic enzyme-linked immunosorbent assay kit for diagnosis of *Borrelia burgdorferi* infection in horses. J Vet Diagn Invest 2008;20(3):321–4.

136. Nicholson WL, Allen KE, McQuiston JH, et al. The increasing recognition of rickettsial pathogens in dogs and people. Trends Parasitol 2010;26(4):205–12.

137. Perille AL, Matus RE. Canine ehrlichiosis in six dogs with persistently increased antibody titers. J Vet Intern Med 1991;5(3):195–8.

138. Bartsch RC, Greene RT. Post-therapy antibody titers in dogs with ehrlichiosis: follow-up study on 68 patients treated primarily with tetracycline and/or doxycycline. J Vet Intern Med 1996;10(4):271–4.

139. Hegarty BC, de Paiva Diniz PP, Bradley JM, et al. Clinical relevance of annual screening using a commercial enzyme-linked immunosorbent assay (SNAP 3Dx) for canine ehrlichiosis. J Am Anim Hosp Assoc 2009;45(3):118–24.

140. Neer TM, Breitschwerdt EB, Greene RT, et al. Consensus statement on ehrlichial disease of small animals from the infectious disease study group of the ACVIM. American College of Veterinary Internal Medicine. J Vet Intern Med 2002;16(3):309–15.

141. Breitschwerdt EB, Hegarty BC, Hancock SI. Doxycycline hyclate treatment of experimental canine ehrlichiosis followed by challenge inoculation with two *Ehrlichia canis* strains. Antimicrob Agents Chemother 1998;42(2):362–8.

142. Harrus S, Kenny M, Miara L, et al. Comparison of simultaneous splenic sample PCR with blood sample PCR for diagnosis and treatment of experimental *Ehrlichia canis* infection. Antimicrob Agents Chemother 2004;48(11):4488–90.

143. Harrus S, Waner T, Aizenberg I, et al. Amplification of ehrlichial DNA from dogs 34 months after infection with *Ehrlichia canis*. J Clin Microbiol 1998;36(1):73–6.

144. Schaefer JJ, Needham GR, Bremer WG, et al. Tick acquisition of *Ehrlichia canis* from dogs treated with doxycycline hyclate. Antimicrob Agents Chemother 2007;51(9):3394–6.

145. Iqbal Z, Rikihisa Y. Reisolation of *Ehrlichia canis* from blood and tissues of dogs after doxycycline treatment. J Clin Microbiol 1994;32(7):1644–9.

146. Wen B, Rikihisa Y, Mott JM, et al. Comparison of nested PCR with immunofluorescent-antibody assay for detection of *Ehrlichia canis* infection in dogs treated with doxycycline. J Clin Microbiol 1997;35(7):1852–5.

147. Matthewman LA, Kelly PJ, Brouqui P, et al. Further evidence for the efficacy of imidocarb dipropionate in the treatment of *Ehrlichia canis* infection. J S Afr Vet Assoc 1994;65(3):104–7.

148. Sainz A, Kim CH, Tesouro MA, et al. Serological evidence of exposure to *Ehrlichia* species in dogs in Spain. Ann N Y Acad Sci 2000;916:635–42.

149. Neer TM, Eddlestone SM, Gaunt SD, et al. Efficacy of enrofloxacin for the treatment of experimentally induced *Ehrlichia canis* infection. J Vet Intern Med 1999;13(5):501–4.

150. Branger S, Rolain JM, Raoult D. Evaluation of antibiotic susceptibilities of *Ehrlichia canis*, *Ehrlichia chaffeensis*, and *Anaplasma phagocytophilum* by real-time PCR. Antimicrob Agents Chemother 2004;48(12):4822–8.

151. Buitrago MI, Ijdo JW, Rinaudo P, et al. Human granulocytic ehrlichiosis during pregnancy treated successfully with rifampin. Clin Infect Dis 1998;27(1):213–5.

152. Krause PJ, Corrow CL, Bakken JS. Successful treatment of human granulocytic ehrlichiosis in children using rifampin. Pediatrics 2003;112(3 Pt 1):e252–3.

153. Schaefer JJ, Kahn J, Needham GR, et al. Antibiotic clearance of *Ehrlichia canis* from dogs infected by intravenous inoculation of carrier blood. Ann N Y Acad Sci 2008;1149:263–9.

154. Littman MP, Goldstein RE, Labato MA, et al. ACVIM small animal consensus statement on Lyme disease in dogs: diagnosis, treatment, and prevention. J Vet Intern Med 2006;20(2):422–34.

155. Huxsoll DL, Hildebrandt PK, Nims RM, et al. Tropical canine pancytopenia. J Am Vet Med Assoc 1970;157(11):1627–32.

156. Barlough JE, Madigan JE, DeRock E, et al. Protection against *Ehrlichia equi* is conferred by prior infection with the human granulocytotropic ehrlichiosis (HGE agent). J Clin Microbiol 1995;33(12):3333–4.

157. Horowitz HW, Aguero-Rosenfeld M, Dumler JS, et al. Reinfection with the agent of human granulocytic ehrlichiosis. Ann Intern Med 1998;129(6):461–3.

158. Davidson DE Jr, Dill GS Jr, Tingpalapong M, et al. Prophylactic and therapeutic use of tetracycline during an epizootic of ehrlichiosis among military dogs. J Am Vet Med Assoc 1978;172(6):697–700.

159. Blagburn BL, Spencer JA, Billeter SA, et al. Use of imidacloprid-permethrin to prevent transmission of *Anaplasma phagocytophilum* from naturally infected *Ixodes scapularis* ticks to dogs. Vet Ther 2004;5(3):212–7.

160. Davoust B, Marie JL, Mercier S, et al. Assay of fipronil efficacy to prevent canine monocytic ehrlichiosis in endemic areas. Vet Parasitol 2003;112(1–2):91–100.

161. Otranto D, Paradies P, Testini G, et al. Application of 10% imidacloprid/50% permethrin to prevent *Ehrlichia canis* exposure in dogs under natural conditions. Vet Parasitol 2008;153(3–4):320–8.

162. Dumler JS, Madigan JE, Pusterla N, et al. Ehrlichioses in humans: epidemiology, clinical presentation, diagnosis, and treatment. Clin Infect Dis 2007;45(Suppl 1): S45–51.

163. Bakken JS, Dumler S. Human granulocytic anaplasmosis. Infect Dis Clin North Am 2008;22(3):433–48.

164. Perez M, Bodor M, Zhang C, et al. Human infection with *Ehrlichia canis* accompanied by clinical signs in Venezuela. Ann N Y Acad Sci 2006;1078:110–7.

Canine Babesiosis

Peter J. Irwin, BVetMed, PhD, FACVSc

KEYWORDS

- *Babesia* • *Theileria* • Piroplasm • Dog • Canine

Canine babesiosis is a clinically significant and geographically widespread hemopro-tozoan disease of domesticated dogs and wild canids. Although the term babesiosis encompasses only species of the genus *Babesia*, it is increasingly apparent from recent studies that parasites of the closely related genus *Theileria* are also capable of infecting dogs. Intraerythrocytic parasites of these 2 genera are collectively referred to as piroplasms because of the round to pear-shaped appearance under light micros-copy; hence the term piroplasmosis is used frequently in this article. Based on their relative sizes, these parasites are broadly divided into 2 groups, large and small piro-plasms (**Figs. 1** and **2**).[1] Although all large forms reported to date belong to the genus *Babesia*, the distinction between small *Babesia* spp and *Theileria* spp cannot be made by microscopic examination alone, necessitating DNA-based molecular techniques for accurate identification.

TAXONOMY AND GEOGRAPHIC DISTRIBUTION

At the time of writing this article there are 12 piroplasm species reported in dogs world-wide (**Tables 1** and **2**). Some of these (see **Table 2**) have been detected by molecular techniques (polymerase chain reaction [PCR]) only, and neither the clinical signifi-cance nor the natural biology of these infections is currently understood.[5,9–11] For the remaining 8 species that have been visualized microscopically and for which there have been clinical descriptions, some (eg, *Babesia canis* [sensu lato], *Babesia conra-dae*, *Babesia gibsoni*) have reasonably well-described geographic distributions. In contrast, the distribution, epidemiology, and disease associations of more recently discovered species remain to be elucidated.[4,7,12]

The United States

In the United States, *Babesia canis vogeli* and *B gibsoni* are the most common and well-documented piroplasm infections.[13] *Babesia vogeli*, a large piroplasm, is trans-mitted by the brown dog tick (*Rhipicephalus sanguineus*), which is adapted to warmer climates. Therefore most reports of *B vogeli* infections come from the southern and southeastern states and from California, where it is well recognized as a problem when large numbers of dogs are confined together, such as in shelters and greyhound

Department of Veterinary Clinical Science, School of Veterinary and Biomedical Sciences, Murdoch University, South Street, Murdoch, Western Australia 6150, Australia
E-mail address: P.Irwin@murdoch.edu.au

Vet Clin Small Anim 40 (2010) 1141–1156
doi:10.1016/j.cvsm.2010.08.001
0195-5616/10/$ – see front matter © 2010 Elsevier Inc. All rights reserved.

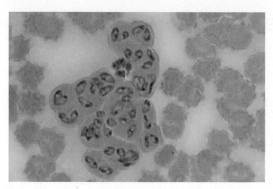

Fig. 1. Large piroplasms (*B vogeli*). This image shows a cluster of infected red cells with typical intraerythrocytic parasites (trophozoites) and free forms (merozoites) (Giemsa, original magnification ×1000).

kennels.[13] In pups, *B vogeli* causes severe babesiosis, yet in adult dogs the clinical signs are often mild.[14] In some dogs that are immunocompromised through concurrent infection, neoplastic disease, or immunosuppressive treatments, *B vogeli* may represent an incidental finding.[15] In recent years, a second large *Babesia* sp resembling *B vogeli* has been reported in immunocompromised dogs, many of which had been splenectomized, in North Carolina, New Jersey, and New York[5,6,8] and most recently in a dog residing in Texas.[16] As many of these dogs had travel histories, it is possible that they were infected in other states throughout southeast United States.

Since its first report in the United States in 1979,[17] *B gibsoni* infection (a small piroplasm, see **Fig. 2**) has gained a certain notoriety as an emerging disease among certain breeds of dogs, notably the American pit bull and Staffordshire terriers[18,19] used for illegal fighting, with occasional reports in other breeds, some of which had been bitten by a pit bull–type dog previously.[18] In western United States, *B conradae* is a small parasite that is closely related to the piroplasm species found in bighorn

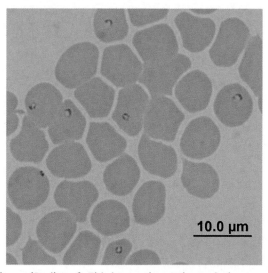

Fig. 2. Small piroplasms (*B gibsoni*). This image shows the typical appearance of small piroplasm species (Giemsa, original magnification ×1000).

Table 1
Geographic distribution of morphologically confirmed piroplasm species of domestic dogs

Size	Species	Synonyms	Vector	Geographic Distribution	Comments and Recent References
Small	Babesia gibsoni	B gibsoni Asia strain	Haemaphysalis longicornis, Haemaphysalis bispinosa Rhipicephalus sanguineus?	Asia and emerging disease worldwide	Outside Asia B gibsoni infection is associated with pit bull terriers and other fighting dogs
	Babesia conradae	B gibsoni (in original reports), Western piroplasm	Unknown	California	Closely related to piroplasms recovered from ungulates and humans[2]
	Babesia microti-like sp	Theileria annae, Spanish isolate/agent	Ixodes hexagonus (putative in Spain)	Northern Spain, eastern Canada and North America	First reported in a dog that had traveled to Spain,[3] recently reported in the United States[4] and Croatia[5] and in foxes[23]
Large	Babesia vogeli	Babesia canis vogeli	R sanguineus	Worldwide, tropical and subtropical climates	Emerging disease in northern and eastern Europe
	Babesia canis	Babesia canis canis	Dermacentor spp	Europe	—
	Babesia rossi	Babesia canis rossi	Haemaphysalis leachi	Sub-Saharan Africa and Southern Africa	—
	Babesia sp	Unnamed large Babesia sp North Carolina isolate	Unknown	East and southeast United States	Immunocompromised dogs[6,7]
	Babesia sp		Unknown	United Kingdom	Single report, 94% genetic similarity with B canis vogeli (18S gene)[8]

Table 2
Piroplasm species detected by molecular diagnostic techniques only, clinical significance unknown

Size	Species	Synonyms	Usual Host	Locations of Reports in Dogs	Comments and References
Small	Theileria sp	Unnamed Theileria sp, South African Theileria sp		South Africa	Closely related to piroplasm recovered from sable antelope[9]
	Theileria annulata		Cattle	Spain (Europe)	[10]
	Theileria equi	Babesia equi	Horse	Spain, Croatia (Europe)	[5,10]
Large	Babesia caballi		Horse	Croatia (Europe)	[5]

sheep, mule deer, and humans and to date has been reported only in California.[2] Before molecular characterization, this organism was thought to be *B gibsoni*,[20,21] which serves to remind us that morphology alone is unreliable in determining the genotype (or species) of a piroplasm. More recently, a *Babesia microti*–like (small) piroplasms, usually reported from Spain,[22] have been identified in blood samples from foxes tested in eastern Canada and North Carolina,[23] and in a female pit bull terrier in Mississippi.[4] It is not known whether this latter finding represents a truly autochthonous (locally acquired) case or whether the parasite gained entry into the Unite States by importation of an infected dog, but the finding that this parasite appears to be prevalent in foxes raises the concerning possibility that this wildlife pool may act as a reservoir for canine infections.

Europe

Canine babesiosis is also of clinical importance in other parts of the world. In Europe, the predominant piroplasm species are *Babesia canis canis* (in central and eastern regions, transmitted by *Dermacentor* ticks), *B vogeli* (in the Mediterranean basin), and *Theileria annae* (in Spain).[1,15,22] However, the custom of traveling with family pets or hunting dogs on recreational trips to distant regions and returning home to places that are well outside the normal enzootic ranges of vector ticks has seen an alarming increase in reports of canine vector-borne pathogens in northern (cooler) regions of mainland Europe and in the United Kingdom, where these diseases were previously unreported.[15,24,25]

Other Regions

In Brazil, South America, *B vogeli* and *B gibsoni* are the canine piroplasms reported.[26,27] Despite sporadic reports, the species of piroplasms and their disease associations are far from clear in many tropical areas of the world, such as in Asia (India, Southeast Asia), Africa, the Caribbean, and the Pacific Island nations, because of the limited research into canine diseases in most of these regions.[28–30] *R sanguineus* is abundant in the warm and humid tropics, and therefore, *B vogeli* is the predominant large babesial species present.[30] For the same reason it has been assumed that *B gibsoni*, the small piroplasm endemic in much of tropical Asia, is also transmitted by this tick species, but convincing experimental data to support this hypothesis are currently lacking. Unlike in the United States and other regions where *B gibsoni* is an emerging infection, it is notable that in much of Asia, *B gibsoni* is not associated with pit bull terrier–type dogs.[30,31] In Japan, *B gibsoni* is endemic and is naturally transmitted by *Haemaphysalis* tick species when not spread by fighting dogs.[32] The most pathogenic form of canine babesiosis is found in the African continent, caused by *Babesia canis rossi* and transmitted by *Haemaphysalis leachi*[33]; both *B vogeli* and *B gibsoni* have each been reported recently in South Africa as well.[34,35]

LIFE CYCLE AND TRANSMISSION

The life cycle is well understood for the *Babesia* species infecting domestic animals. Transmission of sporozoites from the salivary glands of a feeding tick into the subcutaneous tissues and bloodstream of the canine host is the route by which most dogs are infected with canine babesiosis. In the case of *R sanguineus* at least, all 3 stages (larvae, nymphs, and adults) can transmit *B vogeli*.[36] Furthermore, the tick must have been in place for several days before transmission can occur.[36] Once in the host's bloodstream, the parasites invade, feed, and multiply within erythrocytes during repeated phases of asexual reproduction, releasing merozoites that find and invade more red cells. Transmission back to a vector may occur at any time that parasitemia exists; ticks are infected with piroplasms when they take a blood meal from a parasitemic host. After ingestion by the tick, the piroplasms continue to develop by sexual reproduction and maturation, eventually migrating to the cells of the tick's salivary glands in readiness for the next feeding or to its ovaries for transovarial transmission to the next generation of ticks.[37]

Although vector-borne transmission is the natural means by which most pets develop babesiosis, infection has also been reported in neonates as a result of transplacental transmission from the dam[38,39] and by transfusion from an infected blood donor.[40] In addition, the transmission of *B gibsoni* during aggressive interactions between fighting dogs is now recognized as the major route of infection for this species and the reason for its global distribution and clonal expansion.[12,41,42] This is best documented among American pit bull and Staffordshire terriers and Tosa Inu breeds. Although not experimentally proven (for obvious reasons), there now exists plenty of epidemiologic evidence to support dog fighting as a means of viable transmission. It is presumed that the parasites (maybe only very few) are introduced when blood from an infected dog enters the bite wounds of the recipient. There is no evidence that transmission occurs via the saliva from the infected dog. From an epidemiologic perspective, this phenomenon implies that any dog in any country could theoretically be a carrier and a history of being involved in a dogfight with significant bleeding is a risk factor for infection.

PATHOGENESIS OF BABESIOSIS

The severity of babesiosis ranges from subclinical infection to widespread organ failure and death. Most dogs with babesiosis develop hemolytic anemia and/or thrombocytopenia, together with varying degrees of anorexia, fever, splenomegaly, icterus, and pigmenturia. The main determinant of this variable pathogenesis is the species of piroplasm responsible for the infection, but other factors such as the age and immune status of the host and the presence of concurrent infections also influence clinical outcome. The presence of multiple coinfections (as can readily occur when pathogens share the same vector) confounds the attribution of clinical signs to the babesiosis alone.[43] Puppies tend to develop more severe clinical disease than adult dogs, and the unnamed *Babesia* sp in the United States has been reported only in immunocompromised (by cancer or splenectomy) dogs.[8,16] It is not known whether these individuals are inherently more susceptible to the acquisition of infection or whether the parasitemia represents recrudescence of latent infection acquired before splenectomy or tumor development.

The severity of the anemia in babesiosis is not proportional to the degree of parasitemia, which, even in the acute stages of infection, generally remains low. Thus, mechanisms other than direct parasite-induced damage alone have been proposed as the cause of hemolysis in uninfected erythrocytes, including oxidative injury resulting from certain hemolytic toxins[44–46] and immune-mediated mechanisms that result in both intravascular and extravascular hemolysis. In a recent study of naturally acquired babesiosis in Europe, none of the dogs with *B canis canis* infections had erythrocyte membrane-bound immunoglobulins detected by flow cytometry immunophenotyping in contrast with 4 of 6 dogs with *B canis vogeli*,[47] each of which had a regenerative anemia.

Babesiosis is referred to as being complicated or uncomplicated in terms of its pathogenesis.[48] Uncomplicated babesiosis is generally associated with mild to moderate anemia, causing pallor, weakness, icterus, and fever, and varying degrees of pigmenturia (hemoglobinuria and bilirubinuria). Complicated babesiosis refers to pathologic manifestations that cannot be readily explained as a consequence of hemolysis alone and is characterized by dysfunction of one or more organs and a high mortality. This type of babesiosis has been extensively studied in South Africa and is associated with virulent *Babesia rossi*[48] but is increasingly reported in association with serious *Babesia* infections in Europe.[7,49,50] Somewhat paradoxically, hemoconcentration (as opposed to anemia) is reported with some *B rossi* infections and is associated with a high mortality.[51]

Similarities have been noted between complicated canine babesiosis and falciparum malaria in humans.[51,52] Clinicopathologic abnormalities noted in such patients include hypoglycemia, acid-base disturbances, azotemia, and elevations in the levels of liver enzymes and acute phase proteins[53,54] consistent with systemic inflammatory responses leading to multiple organ dysfunction syndrome.[48] The level of C-reactive protein (CRP) is elevated in *B canis* infections and was found to be useful in monitoring the response to antibabesial treatment in naturally infected dogs in a study in Europe,[54] although CRP was not of prognostic value in another study in South Africa.[55] Some of these abnormalities, such as the presence of hypoglycemia (<59.4 mg/dL) at admission, persistent hyperlactatemia (>22.5 mg/dL), and azotemia (elevated serum creatinine levels), have been correlated with a poorer prognosis and increased mortality.[53,56,57] Acute renal failure may complicate some cases of babesiosis; hypoxemia, hemoglobinuric nephropathy, and glomerulonephritis are each considered a mechanism for azotemia and clinical signs of renal insufficiency. Indeed, azotemia has been identified as a risk factor and predictor of mortality in dogs infected with a *Babesia microti*–like agent in northern Spain[57] but is considered an unreliable indicator of renal damage with virulent *B rossi* infections.[58]

CLINICAL SIGNS OF BABESIOSIS

Canine babesiosis may be peracute, acute, or chronic, and the clinical signs vague, including lethargy, weakness, vomiting, anorexia, and fever. More specific signs, such as pale mucous membranes, icterus, splenomegaly, and dark discoloration of the urine, should raise the suspicion of a hemolytic process (**Table 3**). Complicated babesiosis may present with a wide range of unusual and severe clinical signs, including neurologic dysfunction (eg, coma, stupor, and seizures), bleeding diatheses, respiratory failure (pulmonary edema), refractory hypotension, and acute renal failure.[33,53,54] In other cases, it is possible that initial infections may go unnoticed by

Table 3
Differential diagnosis of hemolytic anemia in the dog

Age of Dog	Disorder
Neonates and young dogs	Babesiosis
	Neonatal isoerythrolysis
	Inherited erythrocyte defects (rare)
	Transfusion reactions
Older dogs	Immune-mediated hemolytic anemia
	Babesiosis
	Transfusion reactions
	Heinz body anemia (onion poisoning, drug toxicities)
	Dirofilariasis (caval syndrome)
	Acute zinc and copper toxicosis
	Neoplasia (microangiopathic hemolysis)

the owner or are mild or nonspecific so as not to present for veterinary examination. A chronic phase (referred to as a state of premunition) develops in most cases regardless of whether or not the animal received treatment. The period that an individual can remain an infected carrier is not well studied in dogs, but it is suspected to be for many months, possibly even for life. Chronic infections are often asymptomatic; the dog acts as a carrier of the organism, which may or may not recrudesce at times of stress or immunosuppression.

LABORATORY FEATURES AND THE DIAGNOSIS OF PIROPLASMOSIS

The typical hematologic picture of canine babesiosis is of a regenerative anemia, normal plasma protein levels, a moderate to severe thrombocytopenia, and variable leukocyte abnormalities. However, some dogs with acute babesiosis may have a pre-regenerative anemia,[7,47,51] and veterinarians should recognize that in some chronic cases red cell counts may be normal, although microscopic examination usually reveals mild regenerative features. Many similarities exist between the hematologic features of canine babesiosis and immune-mediated hemolytic anemia; autoagglutination and spherocytosis may be present, and a positive Coombs test result is a common finding in many cases of babesiosis.[51,59] Moderate to severe thrombocytopenia is an extremely common finding; it has been suggested in one study in South Africa that the likelihood of babesiosis was less than 1% in the absence of thrombocytopenia.[60] In a study of subclinical B gibsoni infection in fighting dogs in Japan, it was found that mean platelet counts were significantly lower and antiplatelet IgG levels significantly higher in PCR-positive dogs compared with uninfected dogs.[61] However, overt coagulopathy in canine babesiosis is not common and is found only if there is concurrent disseminated intravascular coagulation or coinfection with other pathogens such as Ehrlichia spp.[43] Mild prolongation of activated partial thromboplastin time, elevation of fibrin degradation product level, and abnormal buccal mucosal bleeding time has been reported in B gibsoni infection.[40]

Serum biochemistry in dogs with babesiosis is generally nonspecific, reflecting the related hypoxemia and hemolysis. Typically there are mild to moderate increases in the concentrations of alanine aminotransferase, aspartate aminotransferase, alkaline phosphatase, and bilirubin, and azotemia is frequently noted and may be prerenal or renal in origin.

DIAGNOSIS

The clinical suspicion of babesiosis should be aroused when a dog presents to the veterinarian with any of the clinical signs listed earlier or if anemia or thrombocytopenia is discovered. A history of tick exposure, living in or previous travel to a tick-endemic area, or recent injury from a dogfight should prompt a specific investigation for babesiosis. In temperate climates, there is a seasonal increase in incidence during the spring and summer months,[62] when the tick vectors are more active and abundant, and a decrease in the fall and winter. In tropical and subtropical climates, the incidence of disease is unchanged throughout the year.[30,31]

When the clinical presentation is suggestive of acute or peracute babesiosis, microscopic examination remains the simplest and most accessible diagnostic test for most veterinarians. In acute babesiosis, microscopy is reasonably sensitive for detecting intraerythrocytic piroplasms, provided that the blood films are well prepared and suitably stained. Parasites must be differentiated from artifacts and cell or stain debris and may themselves appear in a variety of atypical morphologic forms influenced by the blood smear and preparation technique (**Fig. 3**). Visual detection of piroplasms confirms the diagnosis and is sufficient to warrant specific treatment in most cases (see later), but the species (or genotype) of the organism cannot be determined by morphology alone; this requires PCR and genomic sequence analysis. In contrast, the detection of chronic and subclinical babesiosis in carrier dogs requires molecular tools because the sensitivity of microscopy in such cases is very low. If babesiosis is confirmed, the veterinarian should consider the possibility of concurrent infection with other vector-borne pathogens, including *Ehrlichia* spp, *Anaplasma* spp, *Bartonella* spp, *Rickettsia* spp, and *Leishmania*,[28,43] and test appropriately.

Despite improvements in laboratory diagnostic methodologies in recent years, there is no testing procedure that offers a 100% certainty of detecting a piroplasmic infection. The combination of serologic testing and PCR is considered to offer the greatest sensitivity; the current recommendation is to screen suspected cases or blood donors initially by serology and subsequently test seronegative dogs with an appropriate piroplasm PCR.[63]

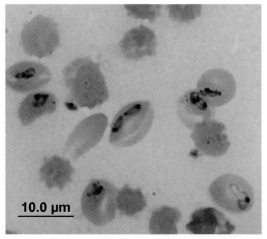

10.0 μm

Fig. 3. Acute *B canis* infection in a pup. Note the crenated erythrocytes and the variation in morphology of the *Babesia* parasites (Giemsa, original magnification ×1000).

Serologic Diagnosis

The immunofluorescent antibody test (IFAT) has been used to diagnose canine babe-siosis since the 1970s.[64–66] Cross-reactions between different piroplasm species have resulted in reduced specificity,[65] and antibodies to some of the more recently described piroplasms may not be detected by conventional IFAT assays,[5,8] resulting in a reduced sensitivity and the potential to overlook infection if only serology is used.

To date, bench-top enzyme-linked immunosorbent assay (ELISA)-based colori-metric tests for in-clinic diagnosis of babesiosis are not available, as they are for canine ehrlichiosis and anaplasmosis, for example, but may be developed for commercial use in the future. Research in this area has been directed toward finding specific immunodominant B gibsoni antigens for use in recombinant protein ELISA.[67–72] Thrombospondin-related adhesive proteins (TRAPs) comprise a group of highly conserved functional proteins identified in apicomplexan parasites that are capable of inducing a host antibody response.[68] An ELISA using recombinant BgTRAP was reported to be more sensitive than other ELISAs using recombinant anti-gens rBgP50, rNgP32, or rBgSA1.[73,74] Recently, a novel antigen (BgP22) has revealed good discrimination between B gibsoni and B canis spp and appears to be useful in detecting chronic B gibsoni infections.[74]

Molecular Diagnosis

The PCR has revolutionized the diagnosis of infectious and parasitic organisms, espe-cially those that are too small to visualize readily or are present in such low numbers as to be beyond the detection limits of conventional methods, such as is the case with the piroplasms. Whereas the detection limit of light microscopy is approximately 0.001% parasitemia, PCR is much more sensitive.[75–77] However, despite its high sensitivity, false-negative PCR results may occur in chronic babesiosis, and it is important to recognize this limitation when screening potential carriers and other asymptomatic dogs such as blood donors.[78]

The ribosomal RNA genes 18S, 5.8S, and 28S and the internal transcribed spacer sequences have been widely used for PCR diagnosis using a variety of techniques; PCR–restriction fragment length polymorphism and nested PCR have been reported to differentiate B vogeli and B gibsoni in a study in Australia[79] and between the large babesial species[75] and B gibsoni in other endemic regions.[80] Further refinement in primer design was reported recently to distinguish between B canis rossi, B canis vogeli, and B canis canis.[81] A study in Japan found that loop-mediated isothermal amplification has advantages of speed and specificity for detecting B gibsoni infec-tions,[82] and reverse line blot hybridization was applied in epidemiologic studies of vector-borne pathogens of dogs and cats in Trinidad[83] and dogs in Africa.[9] Recently, a quantitative fluorescent resonance energy transfer–PCR was developed to differen-tiate Babesia spp by melt curve analysis and applied to blood samples submitted for analysis in the United States and Hong Kong.[31] Some of these PCR methods have been applied to filter paper technologies for ease of transport of samples to distant laboratories and for epidemiologic and other diagnostic studies.[76,79]

TREATMENT

A treatment for piroplasmosis that is 100% safe and efficacious is not available, and most, if not all, dogs treated with specific antibabesial drugs are unlikely to be cured of their infection. A dog in which infection has been confirmed should be regarded as potentially infected for life, despite specific treatment and remission of clinical signs.

Effective management of dogs with piroplasmosis involves both specific and supportive strategies. Supportive treatment is aimed at restoring adequate tissue oxygenation by correction of the anemia, especially if severe, and correction of dehydration and electrolyte disturbances. One or more blood transfusions are indicated to restore and maintain the packed cell volume at a normal value while the specific antiprotozoal drugs start to take effect. In a prospective randomized clinical trial in South Africa, dogs (n = 12) treated with a bovine hemoglobin glutamer (Oxyglobin ® HB-200) had similar improvements in laboratory parameters compared with dogs given transfusions of packed red blood cells, yet the latter had a faster response in their clinical demeanor.[84] As with all anemic animals, fluid therapy should be used judiciously and is primarily indicated if the patient is also dehydrated or anorectic. Oxygen therapy in anemic patients is of questionable benefit unless concurrent lung pathology affects respiratory function and oxygen exchange.

Good nursing support (warmth, nutrition) should also be provided. In addition, dogs with tick infestations should be treated immediately on entry into the clinic with a rapid-acting acaricidal agent (eg, fipronil), and individual ticks removed and destroyed if this is feasible; these latter precautions reduce the risk of ticks contaminating the hospital environment.

Specific treatments for piroplasmosis are listed in **Table 4**. The only drug approved in the United States for the treatment of canine babesiosis is imidocarb dipropionate, and issues concerning drug registration exist in many other countries around the world. Controlled studies of antibabesial treatments in dogs have not been reported. Some drugs appear to have greater efficacy against either the large or the small piroplasms, with the possible exception of diminazene.[1] For this reason, it is important to determine the species of piroplasm, or at least determine if it is large or small, at the time of treatment. Imidocarb dipropionate is used primarily to treat large *Babesia* spp infections,[5,14] and diminazene aceturate (Ganaseg, Berenil; not available in the United States) is used widely in Asia for the treatment of *B gibsoni*, although several clinical reports have raised doubts about its efficacy.[31,34,85] Diminazene is also relatively toxic, and severe side effects have been reported following its use.[86]

Since the first report of using atovaquone and azithromycin (in combination) to treat *B gibsoni* infection[87] there has been considerable experience gained in the United States, Europe, South Africa, Asia, and Australia with its use in dogs for this infection.[34,78,88] The combination of atovaquone and azithromycin (see **Table 4**) is a safe treatment that leads to a rapid clinical improvement in dogs with *B gibsoni* infections, but there are also reports of the drugs failing to clear these parasites, especially with repeated doses, and this failure is mooted to be the result of mutations of the organism's *cytochrome b* gene.[86]

Because of the clinical frustrations with treating chronic, recurrent babesiosis or the unavailability of recognized antibabesial drugs in some regions, other drugs, such as clindamycin, metronidazole, and doxycycline, have been tried with varying degrees of success (see **Table 4**).[31,85,89] However, the absence of rigorous posttreatment testing, the paucity of controlled experimental studies, and the ever-present risk of concurrent infections that are undiagnosed mean that the true efficacy of these treatment regimens remains speculative at best.

PREVENTION

Prevention of piroplasmosis requires that dogs be kept free of tick exposure and avoid fighting with other dogs and that any blood transfusions be carefully screened to ensure absence of pathogens. Both imidocarb (at 6 mg/kg) and doxycycline (5 mg/kg

Table 4
Treatment of piroplasmosis

Babesia Type	Drug Name	Recommended Dose	Notes/Comments
Large	Imidocarb dipropionate	5–7 mg/kg SC or IM once and repeat in 14 d	Pain at site of injection, and nodule may develop at site of injection. Cholinergic signs controlled with atropine (0.05 mg/kg SC)
	Trypan blue	10 mg/kg IV once	Tissue irritant, used as 1% solution. Reversible staining of body tissues occurs. Used in South Africa for *B rossi* infection
Large and Small	Phenamidine isethionate	15 mg/kg SC once, or repeat in 24 h	Nausea, vomiting, and CNS signs are common side effects
	Pentamidine isethiorate	16.5 mg/kg IM, repeat 24 h	Variable and unpredictable toxicity. CNS signs may be severe
	Diminazene aceturate	3.5 mg/kg IM once	Berenil and Ganaseg contain antipyrone
Small	Atovaquone and azithromycin combination	Atovaquone, 13.3 mg/kg PO q 8 h, and azithromycin, 10 mg/kg PO q 24 h, together for 10 d	Mepron contains proguanil, which may induce vomiting in dogs
	Parvaquone	20 mg/kg SC once	—
	Clindamycin	25 mg/kg q 12 h PO	—
	Clindamycin, metronidazole, and doxycycline combination	Clindamycin, 25 mg/kg q 12 h PO, metronidazole, 15 mg/kg PO q 12 h, doxycycline, 5 mg/kg PO q 12 h	—

Abbreviations: CNS, central nervous system; IM, intramuscular; IV, intravenous; PO, by mouth; SC, subcutaneous.

every 24 hours) have been investigated for their prophylactic potential against babe-siosis, yet neither drug has been consistently reliable in this regard. A vaccine for canine babesiosis has been registered in some countries in Europe for nearly 20 years and has shown reasonable efficacy. To date there has been no vaccine available to protect dogs against the other or more recently described piroplasm species.

SUMMARY

Babesiosis continues to pose a threat to dogs worldwide as a cause of anemia, throm-bocytopenia, and a wide variety of clinical signs, ranging from mild, nonspecific illness to peracute collapse and death. Practitioners should be alert to the importance of col-lecting travel and fight history for a patient and should be aware of new piroplasm species that have been described. Asymptomatic infections necessitate careful screening of potential blood donors using a combination of diagnostic testing proce-dures. Current treatment strategies for babesiosis often ameliorate the clinical signs of infection, but these hemoparasites are seldom completely eliminated, and when immunocompromised, recrudescence may occur.

REFERENCES

1. Irwin PJ. Canine babesiosis: from molecular taxonomy to control. Parasit Vectors 2009;2(Suppl 1):1–9.
2. Kjemtrup AM, Wainwright K, Miller M, et al. *Babesia conradae*, sp. Nov., a small canine *Babesia* identified in California. Vet Parasitol 2006;138:103–11.
3. Zahler M, Rinder H, Schein E, et al. Detection of a new pathogenic *Babesia microti*-like species in dogs. Vet Parasitol 2000;89:241–8.
4. Yeagley TJ, Reichard MV, Hempstead JE, et al. Detection of *Babesia gibsoni* and the canine small *Babesia* 'Spanish isolate' in blood samples obtained from dogs confiscated from dogfighting operations. J Am Vet Med Assoc 2009;235(5): 535–9.
5. Beck R, Vojta L, Mrljak V, et al. Diversity of *Babesia* and *Theileria* species in symp-tomatic and asymptomatic dogs in Croatia. Int J Parasitol 2009;39:843–8.
6. Birkenheuer AJ, Neel J, Ruslander D, et al. Detection and molecular characteriza-tion of a novel large *Babesia* species in a dog. Vet Parasitol 2004;124:151–60.
7. Sikorski LE, Birkenheuer AJ, Holowaychuk MK, et al. Babesiosis caused by a large *Babesia* species in 7 immunocompromised dogs. J Vet Intern Med 2010;24(1):127–31.
8. Holm LP, Kerr MG, Trees AJ, et al. Fatal babesiosis in an untravelled British dog. Vet Rec 2006;159:179–80.
9. Matjila PT, Leisewitz AL, Ooshuizen MC, et al. Detection of a *Theileria* species in dogs in South Africa. Vet Parasitol 2008;157:34–40.
10. Criado-Fornelio A, Martinez-Marcos A, Buling-Saraña A, et al. Molecular studies on *Babesia, Theileria* and *Hepatozoon* in southern Europe. Part I: epizootiological aspects. Vet Parasitol 2003;113:189–201.
11. Criado A, Martinez J, Buling A, et al. New data on epizootiology and genetics of piroplasms based on sequences of small ribosomal subunit and cytochrome b genes. Vet Parasitol 2006;142:238–47.
12. Guitian FJ, Camacho AT, Teford SR III. Case-control study of canine infection by a newly recognised *Babesia microti*-like piroplasm. Prev Vet Med 2003;61: 137–45.
13. Boozer AL, Macintire DLK. Canine babesiosis. Vet Clin North Am Small Anim Pract 2003;33:885–904.

14. Irwin PJ, Hutchinson GW. Clinical and pathological findings of *Babesia* infection in dogs. Aust Vet J 1991;68:204–9.

15. Solano-Gallego L, Trotta M, Carli E, et al. *Babesia canis canis* and *Babesia canis vogeli* clinicopathological findings and DNA detection by means of PCR-RFLP in blood from Italian dogs suspected of tick-borne disease. Vet Parasitol 2008;157: 211–21.

16. Holman PJ, Backlund BB, Wilcox AL, et al. Detection of a large unnamed *Babesia* piroplasm originally identified in dogs in North Carolina in a dog with no history of travel to that state. J Am Vet Med Assoc 2009;235(7):851–4.

17. Anderson JF, Magnarelli LA, Donner CS, et al. Canine *Babesia* new to North America. Science 1979;204:1431–2.

18. Birkenheuer AJ, Correa MT, Levy MG, et al. Geographic distribution of babesiosis among dogs in the United States and association with dog bites: 150 cases (2000–2003). J Am Vet Med Assoc 2005;227:942–7.

19. Macintire DK, Boudreaux MK, West GD, et al. *Babesia gibsoni* infection among dogs in the southeastern United States. J Am Vet Med Assoc 2002;220(3):325–9.

20. Conrad P, Thomford J, Yamane I, et al. Hemolytic anemia caused by *Babesia gibsoni* infections in dogs. J Am Vet Med Assoc 1991;199:601–5.

21. Kjemtrup AM, Conrad PA. A review of the small canine piroplasms from California: *Babesia conradae* in the literature. Vet Parasitol 2006;138(1–2):112–7.

22. Camacho AT, Pallas E, Gestal JJ, et al. Infection of dogs in north-west Spain with a *Babesia microti*-like agent. Vet Rec 2001;149:552–5.

23. Birkenheuer AJ, Horney B, Bailey M, et al. Babesia microti-like infections are prevalent in North American foxes. Vet Parasitol 2010;172:179–82.

24. Trotz-Williams LA, Trees AJ. Systematic review of the distribution of the major vector-borne parasitic infections in dogs and cats in Europe. Vet Rec 2003; 152:97–105.

25. Daugschies A. [Import of parasites by tourism and trading]. Dtsch Tierarztl Wochenschr 2001;108:348–52 [in German].

26. Dantas-Torres F, Figueredo LA. Canine babesiosis: a Brazilian perspective. Vet Parasitol 2006;141:197–203.

27. Trapp SM, Messick JB, Vidotto O, et al. *Babesia gibsoni* genotype Asia in dogs from Brazil. Vet Parasitol 2006;141:177–80.

28. Yabsley MJ, McKibben J, Macpherson CN, et al. Prevalence of *Ehrlichia canis, Anaplasma platys, Babesia canis vogeli, Hepatozoon canis, Bartonella vinsonii berkhoffi* and *Rickettsia* spp. in dogs from Grenada. Vet Parasitol 2008;151: 279–85.

29. Suksawat J, Xuejie Y, Hancock SI, et al. Serologic and molecular evidence of coinfection with multiple vector-borne pathogens in dogs from Thailand. J Vet Intern Med 2001;15:453–62.

30. Irwin PJ, Jefferies R. Arthropod-transmitted diseases of companion animals in Southeast Asia. Trends Parasitol 2004;20(1):27–34.

31. Wang C, Ahlowalia SK, Li Y, et al. Frequency and therapy monitoring of canine *Babesia* spp. infection by high-resolution melting curve quantitative FRET-PCR. Vet Parasitol 2010;168:11–8.

32. Miyama T, Sakata Y, Shimada Y, et al. Epidemiological survey of *Babesia gibsoni* infection in dogs in Eastern Japan. J Vet Med Sci 2005;67(5):467–71.

33. Lobetti RG. Canine babesiosis. Comp Cont Ed Pract Vet 1998;20:418–31.

34. Matjila PT, Penzhorn BL, Leisewitz AL, et al. Molecular characterisation of *Babesia gibsoni* infection from a Pit-bull terrier pup recently imported into South Africa. J S Afr Vet Assoc 2007;78(1):2–5.

35. Matjila PT, Penzhorn BL, Bekker CPJ, et al. Confirmation of the presence of *Babesia canis vogeli* in domestic dogs in South Africa. Vet Parasitol 2004;122: 119–25.

36. Shortt HE. *Babesia canis*: the life cycle and laboratory maintenance of its arthropod and mammalian hosts. Int J Parasitol 1973;3:119–48.

37. Mehlhorn H, Schein E. The piroplasms: life cycle and sexual stages. Adv Parasitol 1984;23:370–403.

38. Fukumoto S, Suzuki H, Igarashi I, et al. Fatal experimental transmission of *Babesia gibsoni* infection in dogs. Int J Parasitol 2005;35:1031–5.

39. Taboada J. Babesiosis. In: Greene CE, editor. Infectious diseases of the dog and cat. Philadephia: WB Saunders; 1996. p. 473–81.

40. Stegeman JR, Birkenheuer AJ, Kruger JM, et al. Transfusion-associated *Babesia gibsoni* infection in a dog. J Am Vet Med Assoc 2003;222:959–63.

41. Jefferies R, Ryan UM, Jardine J, et al. Blood, bull terriers and babesiosis: further evidence for direct transmission of *Babesia gibsoni* in dogs. Aust Vet J 2007;85: 459–63.

42. Bostrom B, Wolf C, Greene C, et al. Sequence conservation in the rRNA first internal transcribed spacer region of *Babesia gibsoni* genotype Asia isolates. Vet Parasitol 2008;152:152–7.

43. Kordick SK, Breitschwerdt EB, Hegarty BC, et al. Co-infection with multiple tick-borne pathogens in a Walker Hound kennel in North Carolina. J Clin Microbiol 1999;37:2631–8.

44. Ostsuka Y, Yamasaki M, Yamato O, et al. The effect of macrophages on the erythrocytic oxidative damage and the pathogenesis of anemia in *Babesia gibsoni*-infected dogs with low parasitemia. J Vet Med Sci 2002;64:221–6.

45. Kumar A, Varshney JP, Patra RC. A comparative study of oxidative stress in dogs infected with *Ehrlichia canis* with or without concurrent infection with *Babesia gibsoni*. Vet Res Commun 2006;30:917–20.

46. Chaudhuri S, Varshney JP, Patra RC. Erythrocytic antioxidant defence, lipid peroxides level and blood iron, zinc and copper concentrations in dogs naturally infected with *Babesia gibsoni*. Res Vet Sci 2008;85:120–4.

47. Carli E, Tasca S, Trotta M, et al. Detection of erythrocyte binding IgM and IgG by flow cytometry in sick dogs with *Babesia canis canis* or *Babesia canis vogeli* infection. Vet Parasitol 2009;162:51–7.

48. Jacobson LS. The South African form of severe and complicated canine babesiosis: clinical advances 1994–2004. Vet Parasitol 2006;138:126–39.

49. Schetters T, Kleuskens J, Van De Crommert J, et al. Systemic inflammatory responses in dogs experimentally infected with *Babesia canis*: a haematological study. Vet Parasitol 2009;162:7–15.

50. Matijatko V, Kiš I, Torti M, et al. Septic shock in canine babesiosis. Vet Parasitol 2009;162:263–70.

51. Reyers F, Leisewitz AL, Lobetti RG, et al. Canine babesiosis in South Africa – more than one disease. Does this serve as a model for falciparum malaria? Ann Trop Med Parasitol 1998;92:503–11.

52. Clark IA, Jacobson LS. Do babesiosis and malaria share a common disease process? Ann Trop Med Parasitol 1998;92:483–8.

53. Nel M, Lobetti RG, Keller N, et al. Prognostic value of blood lactate, blood glucose and hematocrit in canine babesiosis. J Vet Intern Med 2004;18: 471–6.

54. Matijatko V, Mrljak V, Kiš I, et al. Evidence of an acute phase response in dogs naturally infected with Babesia canis. Vet Parasitol 2007;144:242–50.

55. Köster LS, Van Schoor M, Goddard A, et al. C-reactive protein in canine babesiosis caused by *Babesia rossi* and its association with outcome. J S Afr Vet Assoc 2009;80(2):87–91.

56. Welzl C, Leisewitz AL, Jacobson LS, et al. Systemic inflammatory response syndrome and multiple organ damage/dysfunction in complicated babesiosis. J S Afr Vet Assoc 2001;72:158–62.

57. Camacho AT, Guitian FJ, Pallas E, et al. Azotaemia and mortality among *Babesia-microti*-like infected dogs. J Vet Intern Med 2004;18:141–6.

58. De Scally MP, Lobetti RG, Reyers F, et al. Are urea and creatinine values reliable indicators of azotaemia in canine babesiosis? J S Afr Vet Assoc 2004;75(3): 121–4.

59. Inokuma H, Okuda M, Yoshizaki Y, et al. Clinical observations of *Babesia gibsoni* infections with low parasitaemias confirmed by PCR in dogs. Vet Rec 2005;156: 116–8.

60. Kettner F, Reyers F, Miller D. Thrombocytopaenia in canine babesiosis and its clinical usefulness. J S Afr Vet Assoc 2003;74:63–8.

61. Matsuu A, Kawabe A, Koshida Y, et al. Incidence of canine *Babesia gibsoni* infection and subclinical infection among Tosa dogs in Aomori Prefecture, Japan. J Vet Med Sci 2004;66(8):893–7.

62. Bourdoiseau G. Canine babesiosis in France. Vet Parasitol 2006;138:118–25.

63. Wardrup KJ, Reine N, Birkenheuer A, et al. Canine and feline blood donor screening for infectious disease. J Vet Intern Med 2005;19:135–42.

64. Anderson JF, Magnarelli LA, Sulzer AJ. Canine babesiosis: indirect fluorescent antibody test for a North American isolate of *Babesia gibsoni*. Am J Vet Res 1980;41:2102–5.

65. Levy MG, Breitschwerdt EB, Moncol DJ. Antibody activity to *Babesia canis* in dogs in North Carolina. Am J Vet Res 1987;48:339–41.

66. Yamane I, Thomford JW, Gardner IA, et al. Evaluation of the indirect immunofluorescent antibody test for diagnosis of *Babesia gibsoni* infections in dogs. Am J Vet Res 1993;54(10):1579–84.

67. Aboge GO, Jia H, Terkawi MA, et al. A novel 57-kDa merozoite protein of *Babesia gibsoni* is a prospective antigen for diagnosis and serosurvey of canine babesiosis by enzyme-linked immunosorbent assay. Vet Parasitol 2007;149:85–94.

68. Zhou J, Fukumoto S, Jia H, et al. Characterization of the *Babesia gibsoni* P18 as a homologue of thrombospondin related adhesive protein. Mol Biochem Parasitol 2006;148:190–8.

69. Jia H, Zhou J, Ikadai H, et al. Identification of a novel gene encoding a secreted antigen 1 of *Babesia gibsoni* and evaluation of its use in serodiagnosis. Am J Trop Med Hyg 2006;75:843–50.

70. Aboge GO, Jia H, Kuriki K, et al. Molecular characterization of a novel 32-kDa merozoite antigen of *Babesia gibsoni* with a better diagnostic performance by enzyme-linked immunosorbent assay. Parasitology 2007;134:1185–94.

71. Zhou J, Jia H, Nishikawa Y, et al. *Babesia gibsoni* rhoptry-associated protein 1 and its potential use as a diagnostic antigen. Vet Parasitol 2007;145:16–20.

72. Goo Y, Jia H, Aboge GO, et al. *Babesia gibsoni*: serodiagnosis of infection in dogs by an enzyme-linked immunosorbent assay with recombinant BgTRAP. Exp Parasitol 2008;118:555–60.

73. Konishi K, Sakata Y, Miyazaki N, et al. Epidemiological survey of *Babesia gibsoni* infection in dogs in Japan by enzyme-linked immunosorbent assay using *B. gibsoni* thrombospondin-related adhesive protein antigen. Vet Parasitol 2008; 155:204–8.

74. Goo Y, Jia H, Terkawi M, et al. *Babesia gibsoni*: identification, expression, localization, and serological characterization of a *Babesia gibsoni* 22-kDa protein. Exp Parasitol 2009;123:273–6.

75. Zahler M, Schein E, Rinder H, et al. Characteristic genotypes discriminate between *Babesia canis* isolates of differing vector specificity and pathogenicity in dogs. Parasitol Res 1998;84:544–88.

76. Tani H, Tada Y, Sasai K, et al. Improvement of DNA extraction method for dried blood spots and comparison of four methods for detection of *Babesia gibsoni* (Asian genotype) infection in canine blood samples. J Vet Med Sci 2008;70: 461–7.

77. Matsuu A, Ono S, Ikadai H, et al. Development of a SYBR green real-time polymerase chain reaction assay for quantitative detection of *Babesia gibsoni* (Asian genotype) DNA. J Vet Diagn Invest 2005;17:569–73.

78. Jefferies R, Ryan UM, Jardine J, et al. *Babesia gibsoni*: detection during experimental infections and after combined atovaquone and azithromycin therapy. Exp Parasitol 2007;117:115–23.

79. Jefferies R, Ryan U, Irwin P. PCR-RFLP for the detection and differentiation of the canine piroplasm species and its use with filter paper-based technologies. Vet Parasitol 2007;144:20–7.

80. Birkenheuer AJ, Levy MG, Breitschwerdt EB. Development and evaluation of a seminested PCR for detection and differentiation of *Babesia gibsoni* (Asian genotype) and *B. canis* DNA in canine blood samples. J Clin Microbiol 2003; 41:4172–7.

81. Duarte SC, Linhares GFC, Romanowsky TN, et al. Assessment of primers designed for the subspecies-specific discrimination among *Babesia canis canis*, *Babesia canis vogeli* and *Babesia canis rossi* by PCR assay. Vet Parasitol 2008;152:16–20.

82. Ikadai H, Tanaka H, Shibahara N, et al. Molecular evidence of infections with *Babesia gibsoni* parasites in Japan and evaluation of the diagnostic potential of a loop-mediated isothermal amplification method. J Clin Microbiol 2004;42: 2465–9.

83. Georges K, Ezeokoli CD, Newaj-Fyzul A, et al. The application of PCR and reverse line blot hybridization to detect arthropod-borne haemopathogens of dogs and cats in Trinidad. Ann N Y Acad Sci 2008;1149:196–9.

84. Zambelli AB, Leisewitz AL. A prospective, randomized comparison of oxyglobin (HB-200) and packed red blood cell transfusion for canine babesiosis. J Vet Emerg Crit Care 2009;19(1):102–12.

85. Susuki K, Wakabyashi H, Takahashi M, et al. A possible treatment strategy and clinical factors estimate the treatment response in *Babesia gibsoni* infection. J Med Sci 2007;69:563–8.

86. Sakuma M, Setoguchi A, Endo Y. Possible emergence of drug-resistant variants of *Babesia gibsoni* in clinical cases treated with atovaquone and azithromycin. J Vet Intern Med 2009;23(3):493–8.

87. Birkenheuer AJ, Levy MG, Breitschwerdt EB. Efficacy of combined atovaquone and azithromycin for therapy of chronic *Babesia gibsoni* (Asian genotype) infections in dogs. J Vet Intern Med 2004;18:494–8.

88. Trotta M, Carli E, Novari G, et al. Clinicopathological findings, molecular detection and characterization of *Babesia gibsoni* infection in a sick dog in Italy. Vet Parasitol 2009;165:318–22.

89. Wulsanari R, Wijaya A, Ano H, et al. Clindamycin in the treatment of *Babesia gibsoni* infections in dogs. J Am Anim Hosp Assoc 2003;114:253–65.

Feline Hemotropic Mycoplasmas

Jane E. Sykes, BVSc (Hon), PhD

KEYWORDS

- *Haemobartonella* • Anemia • Feline immunodeficiency virus
- Feline leukemia virus • Polymerase chain reaction • Zoonosis

Hemotropic mycoplasmas (hemoplasmas) are small (0.3–0.8 μm), unculturable epierythrocytic bacteria that can cause severe hemolytic anemia. These organisms infect a variety of mammalian species and are distributed worldwide. The organism causing disease in cats was previously known as *Haemobartonella felis*, and the disease is referred to as feline infectious anemia. Sequence analysis of the 16S rRNA genes of *Haemobartonella* spp has shown that they belong to a group of fastidious mycoplasmas.[1–3] Over the last 2 decades, the development and application of molecular genetic tests for these organisms had led to a greatly improved understanding of the hemoplasma epidemiology and pathogenesis. Several new hemoplasma species have been discovered in cats, which appear to vary in their pathogenicity, responsiveness to antimicrobial drugs, and ability to form a carrier state.[4–6]

ETIOLOGY AND EPIDEMIOLOGY

Organisms associated with the surface of the feline erythrocyte were first identified in South Africa in 1942, in an anemic cat, and were named *Eperythrozoon felis*.[7] Approximately 10 years later, similar organisms were recognized in cats in the United States in Colorado, and intraperitoneal injection of blood from an infected anemic cat into research cats resulted in anemia in the inoculated cats.[8] In 1955, based on their morphology, the name *Haemobartonella felis* was suggested for the organisms.[9,10] The infection was recognized in cats from other US states[11,12] and several other countries worldwide.[13–23]

With the advent of polymerase chain reaction (PCR) assays in the 1990s, amplification of DNA from *Haemobartonella* spp and *Eperythrozoon* spp became possible. Sequence information from amplified 16S rRNA gene DNA revealed the close similarity of these organisms to mycoplasmas, and *Haemobartonella felis* was renamed *Mycoplasma haemofelis* (Mhf).[2] Around the same time, another epierythrocytic organism was detected in California in a cat that was coinfected with feline leukemia virus (FeLV). This organism was approximately half the size of Mhf, and much less

Department of Medicine & Epidemiology, University of California, Davis, 2108 Tupper Hall, Davis, CA 95616, USA
E-mail address: jesykes@ucdavis.edu

Vet Clin Small Anim 40 (2010) 1157–1170
doi:10.1016/j.cvsm.2010.07.003   vetsmall.theclinics.com
0195-5616/10/$ – see front matter © 2010 Elsevier Inc. All rights reserved.

pathogenic.[4] Initially referred to as the small form, or California variant of *Haemobartonella felis*, the name "*Candidatus* Mycoplasma haemominutum" (Mhm) was subsequently given to this organism (the "*Candidatus*" term for newly described hemoplasmas is required for taxonomy purposes because the organisms cannot be cultured, and will be removed when more information becomes available to support their classification).

Three years later, a third hemoplasma, "*Candidatus* Mycoplasma turicensis" (Mtc), was identified in Switzerland (Latin, *Turicum*, Zurich).[5] This organism has subsequently been reported from Australia, Brazil, Canada, Germany, Italy, Japan, South Africa, United Kingdom, and United States.[24-32] Mtc was discovered using PCR, and has never been identified on blood smears using cytologic examination. In one study, inoculation of 2 specific pathogen-free cats with this organism resulted in mild anemia in one cat and severe anemia in the other, although the cat with severe anemia was also immunosuppressed with glucocorticoids.[5] The same isolate caused mild anemia in 3 additional glucocorticoid-treated cats in a separate study, and the degree of anemia was proportional to the organism load inoculated.[33] Mtc has also failed to cause anemia when inoculated into specific pathogen-free cats.[33,34] Circulating organism loads in cats infected with Mtc, as determined using quantitative PCR assays, have typically been very low.[24,25,33,34] Inoculation of Mtc into research cats was followed by a sharp decline in organism numbers around day 40 post inoculation, and all cats became negative by day 45 post inoculation.[34] Intermittent low-level positive PCR results were detected at later time points in some cats, suggesting that complete elimination of the organism had not occurred. In another study, spontaneous clearance of infection occurred at 10 to 21 weeks post inoculation.[33]

MYCOPLASMA HAEMOFELIS

Using cytologic evaluation of blood smears, Mhf appears as cocci to small (0.6 μm) rings and rods, sometimes forming short chains of 3 to 6 organisms. In most epidemiologic studies that use PCR to detect infection, Mhf is the least prevalent of the 3 feline hemoplasmas, being found in 0.5% to 6% of sick cats visiting veterinary hospitals, although in a few geographic locations Mtc is less prevalent (**Fig. 1**).[24-30,32,35] Experimental inoculation of cats with Mhf results in moderate to severe anemia, and cats infected with Mhf sometimes demonstrate fluctuations in organism loads over the course of infection, with peak organism numbers correlating with dramatic declines in the hematocrit.[4,34,36,37] Young cats may be more susceptible to infection and disease.[27,34]

"*CANDIDATUS* MYCOPLASMA HAEMOMINUTUM"

Most infections with Mhm are chronic and not associated with anemia or other clinical abnormalities. Mhm can be detected using PCR in as many as one-fifth to one-half of cats visiting veterinary hospitals for a variety of reasons, with the prevalence of infection generally increasing with age.[24-30,32,35,38] Inoculation of cats with Mhm can initially be followed by a mild decrease in hematocrit, but the hematocrit generally normalizes after 4 to 6 weeks.[34,36] After infection, organism numbers (as determined using quantitative PCR assays) gradually increase, then reach a plateau.[36] The prevalence of infection in anemic cats has been the same, or lower than the prevalence of infection in nonanemic cats, implying that infection with Mhm is not associated with anemia.[6,24,38,39] Furthermore, inoculation of glucocorticoid-treated, splenectomized cats with Mhm was not associated with development of anemia, and subsequent coinfection with *Bartonella henselae* also did not precipitate development of anemia.[40]

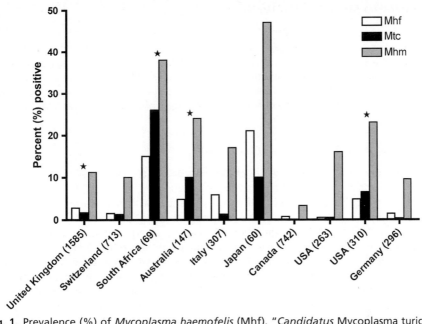

Fig. 1. Prevalence (%) of *Mycoplasma haemofelis* (Mhf), *"Candidatus* Mycoplasma turicensis"* (Mtc), and *"Candidatus* Mycoplasma haemominutum"* (Mhm) when assessed simultaneously in different geographic locations and cat populations worldwide as determined using species-specific PCR assays.[6,24–28,30,32] The presence of a significant number of cats suspected to have hemoplasmosis (based on the presence of anemia or organisms on blood smears) in some of these groups (indicated with a *star*) may have contributed to a high prevalence of infection. The cats from Canada were undergoing wellness examinations; the remaining populations were sick or a mixture of sick and healthy cats.

Nevertheless, there are some suggestions that Mhm may play a role in disease. Case reports have been described of acute hemolytic anemia in pet cats where no apparent causative agent other than Mhm was identified (Sykes, personal observations, 2010),[41–43] although primary immune-mediated hemolytic anemia may have been the underlying cause in some or all of these cats. Cats coinfected with both feline leukemia virus and Mhm develop more significant anemia than cats infected with Mhm alone.[44] Also, cats that are coinfected with FeLV and Mhm may be more likely to develop myeloproliferative disease than are cats infected with FeLV alone.[44] Proposed mechanisms have included immunosuppression induced by the hemoplasma infection, erythroid hyperplasia, and immune stimulation leading to an enhanced rate of mutation and resultant myeloproliferative disease. Infection with Mhm was more prevalent in cats suspected to have hemoplasmosis (generally as a result of acute anemia) than in cats that were sick for a variety of other reasons from a similar geographic location, suggesting a causative role for Mhm in anemia.[27] In addition, among anemic cats, infection with Mhm was associated with higher mean corpuscular volume values than in cats not infected with hemoplasmas, suggesting the possibility of induction of increased erythrocyte turnover by this organism. It is possible that different strains of Mhm exist that vary in their ability to cause anemia, although further research is required to document this proposal.

"CANDIDATUS MYCOPLASMA TURICENSIS"

The prevalence of infection with Mtc in the cat population is similar to that of Mhf, with most studies showing a prevalence of 0.5% to 10% in sick cats visiting veterinary hospitals (see **Fig. 1**).[24–32] The pathogenic potential of Mtc also appears to be low,[24,27,34] although it has induced mild anemia following experimental inoculation of a small number of cats.[5,33] Cofactors, such as coinfection or concurrent immuno-suppression, may be important in the development of anemia in cats infected with Mtc.

RISK FACTORS AND MODE OF TRANSMISSION

Feline hemoplasma infection has been repeatedly and strongly associated with male sex, nonpedigree status, and access to the outdoors.[4,24,25,27,32,38,45,46] In one study from the United States, nearly 90% of cats infected with Mhf were male, and cats infected with Mhf were 7 more likely to be male than uninfected cats.[27] Some studies,[6,27,30,32,35,45,47,48] but not others,[24] have shown an association between retro-virus infection and hemoplasmosis. Cats infected with Mhf in the United States were 6 times more likely to be infected with feline immunodeficiency virus (FIV) than cats negative for hemoplasmas.[27] In Brazil, retrovirus infection was associated primarily with Mhm infection, the association being especially strong for infection with FIV.[35] In Germany, an association with FeLV infection was detected.[32] Coinfections with Mhm and Mtc or Mhm and Mhf have also been recognized.[6,24–28,30,32,38,39,46,49]

The mode of transmission for the feline hemoplasmas has long been an enigma. Fleas have been suggested to transmit Mhf,[47,50] but infection can be widespread in some regions where flea infestation is uncommon.[39] Fleas collected from cats contain hemoplasma DNA, but this is to be expected given their hematophagous activity.[29,51–53] Attempts to use fleas to transmit feline hemoplasmas has been met with disappointing results, with only 1 of 6 inoculated cats developing transient PCR positivity in the absence of illness.[50] Mhf has been detected using PCR in some *Ixodes ricinus* ticks from Europe [54] and Mhm has been detected in unfed *Ixodes ovatus* ticks from Japan.[55] However, studies examining approximately 2000 unfed *Ixodes* spp ticks in Switzerland did not yield evidence of hemoplasma DNA using PCR,[53,56] and infec-tions have been described in suburban areas where there is minimal tick exposure.[6] Geographic variation in the prevalence of hemoplasma infection has been noted in cats, which might support a role for arthropod vectors in transmission.[6,24] All 3 feline hemoplasma species can be detected commonly in wild felids, suggesting the possi-bility that they may act as reservoirs of infection for arthropod transmission.[57] Mosqui-toes have been suggested to play a role in transmission,[6,58] but a recent study of pooled field-caught mosquitoes from Colorado revealed only the DNA of *Mycoplasma wenyonii*, a bovine hemoplasma.[58] Transplacental spread has also been suggested.[59]

The strong male sex predilection and association with retroviral infection has led to renewed interest in the possibility of direct transmission of hemoplasmas through biting and fighting activity. Feline infectious anemia has been observed to occur within weeks of known fighting or biting activities (Sykes, personal observations, 2008). An association with cat-bite abscesses was reported as long as 2 decades ago,[45] although it is possible that these instances represent reactivation of infection following the stress of the fight or bite wound. Hemoplasmas have also been detected in the saliva and feces of experimentally infected cats early in the course of infection, as well as in the saliva, gingival, and claw beds of naturally infected cats, although organism levels in these secretions have been low.[53,60,61] Cats have also become infected through ingestion of approximately 5 mL of infected blood,[10] and so it is possible that the biting animal or the bitten animal may become infected following aggressive activities. Unfortunately, attempts to infect research cats via subcutaneous inoculation of saliva containing Mtc and oral inoculation of 500 μL of Mtc-infected blood were unsuccessful.[33] In contrast, subcutaneous inoculation of as little as 2 drops (10 μL) of Mtc-infected blood led to successful transmission of the organism.[33] Because of the genetic similarity of Mtc to rodent hemoplasmas (*Mycoplasma coccoides* and *Mycoplasma haemomuris*), rodents have been investigated as a potential reservoir of the organism, but to date feline hemoplasma species have not been found in the rodent population.[53] Transmission can occur following blood transfusion, and it is recommended that prospective blood donors be screened for hemoplasma infection using PCR assays.[62]

PATHOGENESIS

After inoculation of experimental cats with Mhf, there is a variable delay of 2 to 34 days before the onset of clinical signs. Cats typically present to veterinarians in this acute phase of disease, which lasts 3 to 4 weeks in the absence of treatment, and is associated with severe anemia and bacteremia. Sharp declines in the hematocrit frequently correlate with the appearance of organisms on blood smears.[4,59] The anemia that occurs may be due to direct damage to the erythrocyte by the organism or through immune-mediated mechanisms, supported by the detection of cold and warm reactive erythrocyte-bound antibodies in infected cats, the cold reactive antibodies appearing earlier in the course of infection.[34,63,64] In one study, such antibodies were only detected in cats infected with Mhf, and not Mhm or Mtc, supporting the higher relative pathogenicity of Mhf.[34] The antibodies were detected shortly after the development of anemia, suggesting insensitivity of the Coombs test early in the course of disease, or the presence of other factors, such as direct organism damage to the erythrocyte, before formation of cold reactive antibodies. Anemia results primarily from extravascular hemolysis, although intravascular hemolysis has been described in some infected cats.[5,43] Increased osmotic fragility and decreased erythrocyte life span have also been noted in cats with hemoplasmosis.[5,63,65-67]

The number of infected erythrocytes, as determined using cytologic examination of blood smears, may decline from 90% to less than 1% in less than 3 hours.[59,64] Recent studies in pigs have suggested that invasion of the erythrocyte cytoplasm by *Mycoplasma suis* may explain organism disappearance during this phase.[67] However, fluctuation in copy numbers of *M haemofelis* as determined using PCR also occurs following infection, which would not be expected if organism disappearance resulted only from invasion of the erythrocyte cytoplasm. Sequestration of the organism in splenic or pulmonary macrophages has been hypothesized as a possible explanation, but there was no evidence of tissue sequestration of Mhf following experimental inoculation of research cats at times when organism copy numbers in the peripheral blood were low.[37]

Provided death does not occur as a result of severe anemia, cats are able to mount an immune response to the infection with a corresponding increase in the hematocrit, and a disappearance of organisms from blood smears. Despite organism disappearance, positive PCR results may persist.[34,68] It has been suggested that recovered cats may remain subclinical carriers for years, the organism evading the host immune system, with possible reactivation of disease with stress, pregnancy, intercurrent infection, or neoplasia.[59,68,69] However, PCR positivity for Mhf is usually associated with the presence of anemia in client-owned cats, and attempts to reproduce disease reactivation experimentally through abscess creation, glucocorticoid or cyclophosphamide administration, and splenectomy have been disappointing.[69] One study showed persistence of positive PCR results for 6 months after recovery from acute infection once antimicrobials were discontinued, and administration of methylprednisolone was associated with reappearance of organisms on blood smears.[68] In contrast to canine hemoplasma infections, for which splenectomy is usually necessary for expression of clinical disease, splenectomy has a variable effect on the course of hemoplasmosis in cats. Reactivation of disease with anemia and cytologically detectable bacteremia has been documented in some chronically infected cats, although other studies suggest splenectomy increases the number of visible organisms in blood smears without causing significant anemia.[64,69] As already noted, infection of splenectomized cats with Mhm does not seem to enhance the pathogenicity of this organism.[40]

CLINICAL SIGNS AND LABORATORY ABNORMALITIES

Listlessness, inappetence or anorexia, and dehydration are common signs of infection with Mhf, and some cats may also present with weight loss. Anemia is manifested by lethargy, mucosal pallor, tachypnea, tachycardia, development of a hemic cardiac murmur, and occasionally syncope or neurologic signs if the anemia is acute and severe. Some owners may report that their cat eats dirt or cat litter, or licks cement. Other physical examination abnormalities may include splenomegaly and, uncommonly, icterus. Some cats may be febrile, and moribund cats may be hypothermic.

The most characteristic abnormality on the complete blood count is a regenerative anemia, with anisocytosis, macrocytosis, reticulocytosis, polychromasia, Howell-Jolly bodies, and occasionally marked normoblastemia. Autoagglutination may be noted in blood smears from some infected cats. Nonregenerative anemia may be noted, either because insufficient time for a regenerative response has elapsed, or as a result of concurrent FeLV infection.[70,71] Concurrent occult infection with hemoplasmas should be considered in any FeLV-positive cat with macrocytosis, even in the absence of reticulocytosis. Anemic cats that are infected with FIV or FeLV should always be tested for concurrent hemoplasma infection, which represents a treatable underlying condition.

White blood cell counts in cats infected with Mhf may be normal, increased, or low. The serum chemistry profile may show increases in alanine aminotransferase activity, hyperbilirubinemia and, uncommonly, prerenal azotemia. Hypoglycemia has also been reported in production animal species infected with hemoplasmas,[72–74] but was not detected in one recent study of experimentally infected cats.[34]

DIAGNOSIS

Differential diagnoses that should be considered for cats presenting with hemoplasmosis are shown in **Box 1**.

Feline hemotropic mycoplasmas cannot be cultured in the laboratory. Cytologic detection of hemoplasmas has very low sensitivity (**Fig. 2**).[36] Mhf is visible using cytologic examination of blood smears less than 50% of the time in cats with acute hemolytic anemia, because organisms may disappear for several days before reappearing on blood smears over the course of infection. It has been recommended that fresh smears be examined, because the organism may detach from erythrocytes in the presence of ethylenediamine tetraacetic acid. When organisms are seen on blood smears, they are usually Mhf.[27] Mtc has never been seen on blood smears. Mhm is generally not visible in chronically infected cats, and although smaller than Mhf, it may be difficult or impossible to distinguish it from Mhf based on size alone.[75] False-positive diagnoses occur commonly when stain precipitate, basophilic

Box 1
Differential diagnosis for cats presenting with anemia due to hemoplasma infection
Primary immune-mediated hemolytic anemia
Feline leukemia virus infection
Feline immunodeficiency virus infection
Feline infectious peritonitis virus infection
Cytauxzoon felis infection
Heinz body hemolytic anemia (zinc, onions, garlic, local anesthetics, propofol, fish)
Pyruvate kinase deficiency
Red cell fragility disorder of Abyssinian and Somali cats
Occult gastrointestinal hemorrhage

stippling, and Howell-Jolly bodies are confused with organisms, so the use of a reputable central veterinary diagnostic laboratory is recommended to confirm the presence of organisms on blood smears.

Diagnostic PCR assays for hemoplasmas have been designed to detect the 16S rRNA gene, and are widely available on a commercial basis through veterinary diagnostic laboratories and veterinary research institutions. These assays are significantly more sensitive than blood smear evaluation, although they may not consistently detect the organism in asymptomatic carrier cats.[4,28,34,36,38,68,76,77] Available assays can be grouped into (1) conventional PCR assays, whereby bands on a gel are interpreted as positive results; and (2) real-time PCR assays, which rely on fluorometric detection of the PCR product, and can provide information regarding organism load. Some conventional PCR assays do not distinguish Mtc from Mhf. Real-time PCR assays are generally species specific, and may be less prone to false-positive results because of

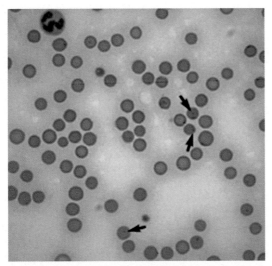

Fig. 2. Romanowsky-stained blood smear showing epierythrocytic bacteria typical of *Mycoplasma haemofelis*. (*Reprinted from* Ettinger SJ, Feldman EC, editors. Veterinary internal medicine expert consult. 7th edition. Saunders; 2009. p. 923; with permission.)

contamination, because tubes are generally not opened in order to detect the PCR product. Occasionally, variant hemoplasma strains may not be detected using real-time PCR assays, resulting in a false-negative test result. Of critical importance when interpreting diagnostic test results is the differing pathogenic potential of each hemoplasma species. Positive test results for any hemoplasma, but especially Mtc and Mhm, do not necessarily imply that these organisms cause a cat's anemia, and other differential diagnoses should always be considered (see **Box 1**). The laboratory must be consulted to determine the species specificity of the assay(s) offered. Dried blood smears can also be used for PCR but are less sensitive than liquid whole blood.[78] Treatment with antimicrobial drugs may result in false-negative results using PCR, so whenever possible, blood must be collected before initiating antimicrobial therapy.

TREATMENT

Before any treatment, diagnostic tests that should be considered include fresh blood smear evaluation, slide agglutination test, complete blood count (including a new methylene blue stain for Heinz bodies), Coombs test, cross-matching and blood typing, serologic tests for FeLV and FIV, a chemistry panel, and urinalysis, as well as PCR testing for Mhf, Mtc, and Mhm. Assays to assess coagulation may also be considered.

Treatment is indicated only for cats with clinical signs and laboratory abnormalities consistent with feline infectious anemia. Treatment of PCR-positive cats that are not anemic (such as those infected with Mhm) is not recommended, because no treatments have yet been identified that eliminate the organism. Mhm does not appear to respond as well as Mhf to therapy with doxycycline or fluoroquinolones, with cats maintaining persistently positive PCR test results in the face of antimicrobial drug therapy.[40,79] Furthermore, those with negative PCR results may not necessarily have completely cleared the infection.[34] Antimicrobial therapy cannot therefore be used to reliably eliminate infection from potential blood donors. Spontaneous clearance of bacteremia may occur in cats infected with Mtc.[24,33,34]

The recommended treatment for hemoplasmosis is doxycycline (10 mg/kg/d, by mouth) for a minimum of 2 weeks. In addition, transfusion with packed red cells or whole blood is indicated if there is severe anemia that is associated with clinical signs such as weakness, tachypnea, or tachycardia. Because of the potential for esophagitis, it has been recommended that administration of doxycycline hyclate be followed by administration of a bolus of several milliliters of water, and ideally a suspension, rather than a tablet, be administered.[80,81] Doxycycline has not been reported to cause yellow discoloration of the teeth in young cats or dogs, and is now considered safe for use in children.[82] Enrofloxacin (5 mg/kg/d, by mouth) is a suitable alternative to doxycycline[83] but has the potential to cause acute retinal damage in cats, so doxycycline is preferred. Where available, pradofloxacin also appears to be a suitable alternative.[84] Azithromycin was ineffective for treatment of hemoplasmosis in cats using an experimental model.[76]

The use of immunosuppressive doses of glucocorticoids to suppress associated immune-mediated damage to erythrocytes is controversial, given that glucocorticoids may cause reactivation of latent infection. The use of glucocorticoids (1 mg/kg by mouth every 12 hours) should be reserved for cats that fail to respond to antimicrobial therapy alone, or for cats in which the diagnosis is uncertain.

Treatment with doxycycline and red blood cell transfusions should be commenced before the results of PCR are available, which is typically within 1 to 3 days. Again, the results of epidemiologic studies suggest that alternative diagnoses should be considered in cats testing positive for Mtc or Mhm, or in cats testing negative for hemoplasmas that fail to respond to antimicrobial therapy.

Hemoplasmas have been shown to survive up to 1 week in stored blood products.[85] Potential blood donor cats should always be screened for Mhf infection using PCR and excluded as blood donors if they test positive. The significance of positive test results for the other 2 hemoplasma species is less clear. Excluding cats testing positive for Mhm presents a difficult situation because the prevalence of infection in the cat population is frequently high, and inoculation of splenectomized, glucocorticoid-treated cats has not been associated with anemia in the authors' studies.[40] However, as noted earlier, strain variation may exist within this species, with some strains being more capable of causing anemia than others. Until more information becomes available regarding the pathogenic potential of this organism, blood testing negative for all hemoplasma species is preferred for transfusion purposes.

PUBLIC HEALTH IMPLICATIONS

Hemotropic organisms that resemble hemoplasmas using cytologic examination of blood smears have occasionally been documented in humans, including anemic patients with acquired immunodeficiency syndrome and systemic lupus erythematosus.[86–89] Recently, *M haemofelis* was detected using PCR in an immunodeficiency virus–infected human from Brazil who was coinfected with *Bartonella henselae*,[90] suggesting that *M haemofelis* may have zoonotic potential. Thus, until more is understood regarding the zoonotic potential of these organisms, caution is advised when handling blood or tissues from infected cats.

SUMMARY

Three species of hemotropic mycoplasmas are known to infect cats worldwide: *M haemofelis*, Mtc, and Mhm. These organisms were previously known as *Haemobartonella felis*, but are now known to be mycoplasmas. *M haemofelis* is the most pathogenic species and causes hemolytic anemia, sometimes with positive Coombs test results, in immunocompetent cats. The pathogenicity of Mtc and Mhm is controversial, as they are frequently detected in nonanemic cats, although they cause mild, transient reduction in the hematocrit for a few weeks following experimental infection. Organisms seen on blood smears are most commonly *M haemofelis* and less commonly Mhm may be seen, although blood smears are unreliable for diagnosis of hemoplasmosis because of their lack of sensitivity and specificity. Assays based on PCR technology are the most sensitive and specific diagnostic tests available for these organisms, because they cannot be cultured in the laboratory. It is important that practitioners understand the clinical significance of a positive test result for each hemoplasma species. Other differential diagnoses for hemolytic anemia should be considered in cats testing positive for Mtc and Mhm, because the presence of these organisms is not always associated with anemia. Blood from infected cats should be handled with care because of the potential zoonotic nature of hemoplasma infections. The treatment of choice for cats with clinical disease is doxycycline.

REFERENCES

1. Rikihisa Y, Kawahara M, Wen B, et al. Western immunoblot analysis of *Haemobartonella muris* and comparison of 16S rRNA gene sequences of *H. muris, H. felis,* and *Eperythrozoon suis.* J Clin Microbiol 1997;35(4):823–9.

2. Neimark H, Johansson KE, Rikihisa Y, et al. Proposal to transfer some members of the genera *Haemobartonella* and *Eperythrozoon* to the genus *Mycoplasma* with descriptions of 'Candidatus *Mycoplasma haemofelis*', 'Candidatus *Mycoplasma haemomuris*', 'Candidatus *Mycoplasma haemosuis*' and 'Candidatus *Mycoplasma wenyonii*'. Int J Syst Evol Microbiol 2001;51(Pt 3):891–9.

3. Johansson KE, Tully JG, Bolske G, et al. *Mycoplasma cavipharyngis* and *Mycoplasma fastidiosum*, the closest relatives to *Eperythrozoon spp.* and *Haemobartonella spp.* FEMS Microbiol Lett 1999;174(2):321–6.

4. Foley JE, Harrus S, Poland A, et al. Molecular, clinical, and pathologic comparison of two distinct strains of *Haemobartonella felis* in domestic cats. Am J Vet Res 1998;59(12):1581–8.

5. Willi B, Boretti FS, Cattori V, et al. Identification, molecular characterization, and experimental transmission of a new hemoplasma isolate from a cat with hemolytic anemia in Switzerland. J Clin Microbiol 2005;43(6):2581–5.

6. Sykes JE, Drazenovich NL, Ball LM, et al. Use of conventional and real-time polymerase chain reaction to determine the epidemiology of hemoplasma infections in anemic and nonanemic cats. J Vet Intern Med 2007;21(4):685–93.

7. Clark R. *Eperythrozoon felis* (sp. nov.) in a cat. J S Afr Vet Med Assoc 1942;13(1):15–6.

8. Flint JC, Moss LC. Infectious anemia in cats. J Am Vet Med Assoc 1953;122(910): 45–8.

9. Flint JC, McKelvie DH. Feline infectious anemia—diagnosis and treatment. In: Proceedings of the American Veterinary Medical Association. Salt Lake City (UT); 1953. p. 240–2.

10. Flint JC, Roepke MH, Jensen R. Feline infectious anemia. II. Experimental cases. Am J Vet Res 1959;20:33–40.

11. Flint JC, Roepke MH, Jensen R. Feline infectious anemia. I. Clinical aspects. Am J Vet Res 1958;19:164–8.

12. Splitter EJ, Castro ER, Kanawyer WL. Feline infectious anemia. Vet Med 1956;51: 17–22.

13. Seamer J, Douglas SW. A new blood parasite of British cats. Vet Rec 1959;71(20): 405–8.

14. Bedford PG. Feline infectious anaemia in the London area. Vet Rec 1970;87(11): 305–10.

15. Manusu HP. Infectious feline anaemia in Australia. Aust Vet J 1961;37:405.

16. Taylor D, Sandholm M, Valtonen M, et al. Feline infectious anemia recognized in Finland. Nord Vet Med 1967;19:277–81.

17. Prieur WD. [Beitrag zur infectiosen Anami der Katze]. Kleint Prax 1960;5:87–9 [in German].

18. Flagstad A, Larsen SA. The occurrence of feline infectious anemia in Denmark. Nord Vet Med 1969;21:129–41.

19. Espada Y, Prats A, Albo F. Feline haemobartonellosis. Vet Int 1991;1:35–40.

20. Bobade PA, Akinyemi JO. A case of haemobartonellosis in a cat in Ibadan. Nig Vet J 1981;10(1):23–5.

21. Maede Y, Hata R, Shibata H, et al. Clinical observation on 6 cases of feline infectious anaemia. J Jap Vet Med Assoc 1974;27:267–72.

22. Anderson DC, Charleston WA. *Haemobartonella felis*. N Z Vet J 1967;15(3):47.

23. Collins JD, Neumann HJ. Feline infectious anaemia: a first case. Irish Vet J 1968; 22:88–90.

24. Willi B, Boretti FS, Baumgartner C, et al. Prevalence, risk factor analysis, and follow-up of infections caused by three feline hemoplasma species in Switzerland. J Clin Microbiol 2006;44(3):961–9.

25. Willi B, Tasker S, Boretti FS, et al. Phylogenetic analysis of 'Candidatus Mycoplasma turicensis' isolates from pet cats in the United Kingdom, Australia, and South Africa, with analysis of risk factors for infection. J Clin Microbiol 2006; 44(12):4430–5.
26. Fujihara M, Watanabe M, Yamada T, et al. Occurrence of 'Candidatus Mycoplasma turicensis' infection in domestic cats in Japan. J Vet Med Sci 2007; 69(10):1061–3.
27. Sykes JE, Terry JC, Lindsay LL, et al. Prevalences of various hemoplasma species among cats in the United States with possible hemoplasmosis. J Am Vet Med Assoc 2008;232(3):372–9.
28. Peters IR, Helps CR, Willi B, et al. The prevalences of three species of feline hemoplasmas in samples submitted to a diagnostics service as determined by three novel real-time duplex PCR assays. Vet Microbiol 2008;126(1–3):142–50.
29. Kamrani A, Parreira VR, Greenwood J, et al. The prevalence of Bartonella, hemoplasma, and Rickettsia felis infections in domestic cats and cat fleas in Ontario. Can J Vet Res 2008;72(5):411–9.
30. Gentilini F, Novacco M, Turba ME, et al. Use of combined conventional and real-time PCR to determine the epidemiology of feline haemoplasma infections in northern Italy. J Feline Med Surg 2009;11(4):277–85.
31. Santos AP, Messick JB, Biondo AW, et al. Design, optimization, and application of a conventional PCR assay with an internal control for detection of 'Candidatus Mycoplasma turicensis' 16S rDNA in domestic cats from Brazil. Vet Clin Pathol 2009;38(4):443–52.
32. Laberke S, Just F, Pfister K, et al. Prevalence of hemoplasma infection in cats in southern Bavaria, Germany, and risk factor analysis. Berl Munch Tierarztl Wochenschr 2010;123(1–2):42–8.
33. Museux K, Boretti FS, Willi B, et al. In vivo transmission studies of 'Candidatus Mycoplasma turicensis' in the domestic cat. Vet Res 2009;40(5):45.
34. Tasker S, Peters IR, Papasouliotis K, et al. Description of outcomes of experimental infection with feline haemoplasmas: copy numbers, haematology, Coombs' testing and blood glucose concentrations. Vet Microbiol 2009; 139(3–4):323–32.
35. Macieira DB, de Menezes Rde C, Damico CB, et al. Prevalence and risk factors for hemoplasmas in domestic cats naturally infected with feline immunodeficiency virus and/or feline leukemia virus in Rio de Janeiro, Brazil. J Feline Med Surg 2008;10(2):120–9.
36. Tasker S, Helps CR, Day MJ, et al. Use of real-time PCR to detect and quantify Mycoplasma haemofelis and 'Candidatus Mycoplasma haemominutum' DNA. J Clin Microbiol 2003;41(1):439–41.
37. Tasker S, Peters IR, Day MJ, et al. Distribution of Mycoplasma haemofelis in blood and tissues following experimental infection. Microb Pathog 2009;47:334–40.
38. Tasker S, Binns SH, Day MJ, et al. Use of a PCR assay to assess the prevalence and risk factors for Mycoplasma haemofelis and 'Candidatus Mycoplasma haemominutum' in cats in the United Kingdom. Vet Rec 2003;152(7): 193–8.
39. Jensen WA, Lappin MR, Kamkar S, et al. Use of a polymerase chain reaction assay to detect and differentiate two strains of Haemobartonella felis in naturally infected cats. Am J Vet Res 2001;62(4):604–8.
40. Sykes JE, Henn JB, Kasten RW, et al. Bartonella henselae infection in splenectomized domestic cats previously infected with hemotropic Mycoplasma species. Vet Immunol Immunopathol 2007;116(1–2):104–8.

41. de Lorimier LP, Messick JB. Anemia associated with '*Candidatus* Mycoplasma haemominutum' in a feline leukemia virus-negative cat with lymphoma. J Am Anim Hosp Assoc 2004;40(5):423–7.

42. Reynolds CA, Lappin MR. '*Candidatus* Mycoplasma haemominutum' infections in 21 client-owned cats. J Am Anim Hosp Assoc 2007;43(5):249–57.

43. Hornok S, Meli ML, Gönczi E, et al. First molecular identification of '*Candidatus* Mycoplasma haemominutum' from a cat with fatal haemolytic anaemia in Hungary. Acta Vet Hung 2008;56(4):441–50.

44. George JW, Rideout BA, Griffey SM, et al. Effect of preexisting FeLV infection or FeLV and feline immunodeficiency virus coinfection on pathogenicity of the small variant of *Haemobartonella felis* in cats. Am J Vet Res 2002;63(8): 1172–8.

45. Grindem CB, Corbett WT, Tomkins MT. Risk factors for *Haemobartonella felis* infection in cats. J Am Vet Med Assoc 1990;196(1):96–9.

46. Luria BJ, Levy JK, Lappin MR, et al. Prevalence of infectious diseases in feral cats in northern Florida. J Feline Med Surg 2004;6(5):287–96.

47. Nash AS, Bobade PA. *Haemobartonella felis* infection in cats from the Glasgow area. Vet Rec 1986;119(15):373–5.

48. Harrus S, Klement E, Aroch I, et al. Retrospective study of 46 cases of feline hae-mobartonellosis in Israel and their relationships with FeLV and FIV infections. Vet Rec 2002;151(3):82–5.

49. Lobetti RG, Tasker S. Diagnosis of feline haemoplasma infection using a real-time PCR assay. J S Afr Vet Assoc 2004;75(2):94–9.

50. Woods JE, Brewer MM, Hawley JR, et al. Evaluation of experimental transmission of '*Candidatus* Mycoplasma haemominutum' and *Mycoplasma haemofelis* by *Ctenocephalides felis* to cats. Am J Vet Res 2005;66(6):1008–12.

51. Shaw SE, Kenny MJ, Tasker S, et al. Pathogen carriage by the cat flea *Ctenoce-phalides felis* (Bouché) in the United Kingdom. Vet Microbiol 2004;102(3–4): 183–8.

52. Lappin MR, Griffin B, Brunt J, et al. Prevalence of *Bartonella* species, haemoplasma species, *Ehrlichia* species, *Anaplasma phagocytophilum* and *Neorickettsia risticii* DNA in the blood of cats and their fleas in the United States. J Feline Med Surg 2006; 8(2):85–90.

53. Willi B, Boretti FS, Meli ML, et al. Real-time PCR investigation of potential vectors, reservoirs, and shedding patterns of feline hemotropic mycoplasmas. Appl Environ Microbiol 2007;73(12):3798–802.

54. Schabereiter-Gurtner C, Lubitz W, Rölleke S. Application of broad-range 16S rRNA PCR amplification and DGGE fingerprinting for detection of tick-infecting bacteria. J Microbiol Methods 2003;52(2):251–60.

55. Taroura S, Shimada Y, Skata Y, et al. Detection of DNA of '*Candidatus* Myco-plasma haemominutum' and *Spiroplasma spp.* in unfed ticks collected from vegetation in Japan. J Vet Med Sci 2005;67(12):1277–9.

56. Willi B, Meli ML, Lüthy R, et al. Development and application of a universal hemo-plasma screening assay based on the SYBR green PCR principle. J Clin Micro-biol 2010;47(12):4049–54.

57. Willi B, Filoni C, Catão-Dias JL, et al. Worldwide occurrence of feline hemoplasma infections in wild felid species. J Clin Microbiol 2007;45(4):1159–66.

58. Lin PC, Hawley JR, Bolling BG, et al. Prevalence of hemoplasma DNA in field-caught mosquitoes in Colorado [abstract]. J Vet Intern Med 2009;23:718.

59. Harvey JW, Gaskin JM. Experimental feline haemobartonellosis. J Am Anim Hosp Assoc 1977;13:28–38.

60. Dean RS, Helps CR, Gruffydd-Jones TJ, et al. Use of real-time PCR to detect *Mycoplasma haemofelis* and '*Candidatus* M. haemominutum' in the saliva and salivary glands of haemoplasma-infected cats. J Feline Med Surg 2008;10(4):413–7.
61. Lappin MR, Dingman P, Levy J, et al. Detection of hemoplasma DNA on the gingival and claw beds of naturally exposed cats [abstract]. J Vet Intern Med 2008;22(3):779.
62. Wardrop J, Reine N, Birkenheuer A, et al. Canine and feline blood donor screening for infectious disease. J Vet Intern Med 2005;19(1):135–42.
63. Zulty JC, Kociba GJ. Cold agglutinins in cats with haemobartonellosis. J Am Vet Med Assoc 1990;196(6):907–10.
64. Alleman AR, Pate MG, Harvey JW, et al. Western immunoblot analysis of the antigens of *Haemobartonella felis* with sera from experimentally infected cats. J Clin Microbiol 1999;37(5):1474–9.
65. Maede Y, Hata R. Studies on feline haemobartonellosis. II. The mechanism of anemia produced by infection with *Haemobartonella felis*. Nippon Juigaku Zasshi 1975;37(1):49–54.
66. Maede Y. Studies on feline haemobartonellosis. IV. Lifespan of erythrocytes of cats infected with *Haemobartonella felis*. Nippon Juigaku Zasshi 1975;37(5):269–72.
67. Groebel K, Hoelzle K, Wittenbrink MM, et al. *Mycoplasma suis* invades porcine erythrocytes. Infect Immun 2009;77(2):576–84.
68. Berent LM, Messick JB, Cooper SK. Detection of *Haemobartonella felis* in cats with experimentally induced acute and chronic infections, using a polymerase chain reaction assay. Am J Vet Res 1998;59(10):1215–20.
69. Harvey JW, Gaskin JM. Feline haemobartonellosis: attempts to induce relapses of clinical disease in chronically infected cats. J Am Anim Hosp Assoc 1978;14:453.
70. VanSteenhouse JL, Taboada J, Dorfman MI. *Haemobartonella felis* infection with atypical hematological abnormalities. J Am Anim Hosp Assoc 1995;31(2):165–9.
71. Bobade PA, Nash AS, Rogerson P. Feline haemobartonellosis: clinical, haematological and pathological studies in natural infections and the relationship to infection with feline leukaemia virus. Vet Rec 1988;122(2):32–6.
72. Love JN, Wilson RP, McEwen EG, et al. Metabolism of [14C] glucose in Haemobartonella-like infected erythrocytes in splenectomized calves. Am J Vet Res 1977;38:739–41.
73. McLaughlin BG, Evans CN, McLaughlin PS, et al. An *Eperythrozoon*-like parasite in llamas. J Am Vet Med Assoc 1990;197:1170–5.
74. Zachary JF, Smith AR. Experimental porcine eperythrozoonosis: T-lymphocyte suppression and misdirected immune responses. Am J Vet Res 1985;46:821–30.
75. Tasker S. Feline haemobartonellosis: lessons from reclassification and new methods of diagnosis. In: Proceedings of the 20th American College of Veterinary Internal Medicine Forum. Dallas (TX); 2002. p. 636.
76. Westfall DS, Jensen WA, Reagan WJ, et al. Inoculation of two genotypes of *Haemobartonella felis* (California and Ohio variants) to induce infection in cats and the response to treatment with azithromycin. Am J Vet Res 2001;62(5):687–91.
77. Messick JB, Berent LM, Cooper SK. Development and evaluation of a PCR-based assay for detection of *Haemobartonella felis* in cats and differentiation of *H. felis* from related bacteria by restriction fragment length polymorphism analysis. J Clin Microbiol 1998;36(2):462–6.
78. Sykes JE, Owens SD, Terry JC, et al. Use of dried blood smears for detection of feline hemoplasmas using real-time polymerase chain reaction. J Vet Diagn Invest 2008;20(5):616–20.

79. Tasker S, Caney SM, Day MJ, et al. Effect of chronic feline immunodeficiency infection, and efficacy of marbofloxacin treatment, on 'Candidatus Mycoplasma haemominutum' infection. Microbes Infect 2006;8(3):653–61.

80. German AJ, Cannon MJ, Dye C, et al. Oesophageal strictures in cats associated with doxycycline therapy. J Feline Med Surg 2005;7(1):33–41.

81. McGrotty YL, Knottenbelt CM. Oesophageal stricture in a cat due to oral administration of tetracyclines. J Small Anim Pract 2002;43(5):221–3.

82. Volovitz B, Shkap R, Amir J, et al. Absence of tooth staining with doxycycline treatment in young children. Clin Pediatr (Phila) 2007;46(2):121–6.

83. Tasker S, Helps CR, Day MJ, et al. Use of a Taqman PCR to determine the response of Mycoplasma haemofelis infection to antibiotic treatment. J Microbiol Methods 2004;56(1):63–71.

84. Dowers KL, Tasker S, Radecki SV, et al. Use of pradofloxacin to treat experimentally induced Mycoplasma haemofelis infection in cats. Am J Vet Res 2009;70(1): 105–11.

85. Gary AT, Richmond HL, Tasker S, et al. Survival of Mycoplasma haemofelis and 'Candidatus Mycoplasma haemominutum' in blood of cats used for transfusions. J Feline Med Surg 2006;8(5):321–6.

86. Puntaric V, Borcic D, Vukelic D, et al. Eperythrozoonosis in man. Lancet 1986; 2(8511):868–9.

87. Duarte MI, Oliveira MS, Shikanai-Yasuda MA, et al. Haemobartonella-like microorganism infection in AIDS patients: ultrastructural pathology. J Infect Dis 1992; 165(5):976–7.

88. Kallick CA, Levin S, Reddi KT, et al. Systemic lupus erythematosus associated with haemobartonella-like organisms. Nat New Biol 1972;236(66):145–6.

89. Archer GL, Coleman PH, Cole RM, et al. Human infection from an unidentified erythrocyte-associated bacterium. N Engl J Med 1979;301(17):897–900.

90. dos Santos AP, dos Santos RP, Biondo AW, et al. Hemoplasma infection in an HIV-positive patient, Brazil. Emerg Infect Dis 2008;14(12):1922–4.

Antifungal Treatment of Small Animal Veterinary Patients

Daniel S. Foy, MS, DVM*, Lauren A. Trepanier, DVM, PhD

KEYWORDS

• Antifungal • Amphotericin B • Azole • Systemic mycoses

The incidence of systemic fungal infections has been increasing in human patients, because of immunosuppression from human immunodeficiency virus infection, hematopoietic stem cell transplants, solid organ transplants, chemotherapy, and hematologic malignancy.[1] Until recently, treatment of systemic mycoses in humans was limited to intravenous (IV) amphotericin B and oral ketoconazole. However, in the last 2 decades, significant progress has been made in the development of first-generation triazole drugs, newer second-generation triazole drugs, and echinocandins.[2] The number of available antifungal agents has increased by 30% since 2000.[2]

Development of safe new antifungal therapies has been constrained by fungal organisms being eukaryotic; many of the potential cellular or mechanistic targets, if disrupted, also cause host toxicity. For example, traditional antifungal medications that target ergosterol, or its production, can cause toxicity in mammalian cells via inhibition of cholesterol production or damage to cell membranes. Newer therapies are being directed at components unique to fungal organisms, thereby sparing mammalian cells.[3] This review discusses the currently available, and most frequently used, antifungal therapies, and the indications for their use in dogs and cats. In addition, newer alternatives, which have recently been approved for use in humans, are briefly reviewed. Although these newer drugs have had limited use to date in veterinary patients because of high cost,[4] some of these products may become more affordable for veterinary use in the near future.

AMPHOTERICIN B

Since its discovery in 1956 and increased availability in the early 1960s, amphotericin B has become, and remains, the reference treatment of invasive fungal infections. Amphotericin B is a macrocyclic polyene antibiotic originally extracted from

The authors have nothing to disclose.
Department of Medical Sciences, School of Veterinary Medicine, University of Wisconsin-Madison, 2015 Linden Drive, Madison, WI 53706, USA
* Corresponding author.
E-mail address: dfoy@svm.vetmed.wisc.edu

Streptomyces nodosus. This drug forms micelles with fungal ergosterol, which creates channels in the fungal membrane, alters cell permeability, and allows leakage of ions and cellular components from the fungal organism.[5] The effectiveness of amphotericin B is because of its greater affinity for ergosterol, the major sterol of fungal cell membranes, compared with cholesterol, the major sterol of mammalian cell membranes.[6]

Amphotericin B is minimally absorbed from the gastrointestinal tract, and effective treatment requires IV administration. The major limiting factor in the use of amphotericin B is cumulative nephrotoxicity[7]; however, the only absolute contraindication to use is anaphylaxis, reported in approximately 1% of treated people.[8] The cause of nephrotoxicity remains incompletely understood, but may be related to both direct toxicity to epithelial cell membranes and renal vasoconstriction, which leads to a reduction in renal blood flow and glomerular filtration rate (GFR).[9–11] Studies in both rats and dogs have suggested that sodium depletion increases, whereas sodium loading reduces, the nephrotoxicity associated with amphotericin B.[10,12] In humans, serum creatinine is monitored during treatment; a clinically significant increase is considered to be a new increase higher than the normal range, or an increase of greater than 20% from the baseline value.[13]

The inherent nephrotoxicity of the original amphotericin B formulation (a dispersion with sodium deoxycholate) led to the development of 3 new formulations: liposomal preparation, lipid complex, and colloidal dispersion with cholesterol sulfate (**Table 1**).[14–16]

Liposomal amphotericin B (lip-amB; AmBisome, Astellas Pharma) was the first of the lipid-incorporated preparations to be marketed. In this formulation, amphotericin B is encapsulated within liposomes composed of hydrogenated soya phosphatidylcholine, cholesterol, and distearoylphosphatidylglycerol, in a 10:5:4 ratio.[17] Lip-amB achieves higher plasma concentrations than the original formulation; this is believed

Table 1
Summary of amphotericin B formulations and approximate cost

Amphotericin B Formulation	Characteristics	Cost
Colloidal dispersion with sodium deoxycholate (original formulation)	Sodium deoxycholate added to enable reconstitution (amphotericin B is insoluble in water)	$35 per 50-mg vial
Liposome encapsulated	Amphotericin B included in a single bilayer liposome Liposomes form in an aqueous environment Lipophilic nature of amphotericin B enables it to become a natural part of the liposome bilayer	$285 per 50-mg vial
Lipid complex (ABLC)	Amphotericin B complexed with 2 phospholipids 1:1 drug/lipid molar ratio Yellow and opaque appearance	$360 per 100-mg vial
Colloidal dispersion with cholesterol sulfate	Amphotericin B stabilized with cholesterol sulfate in a colloidal complex Amphotericin B released and binds to lipoproteins	$240 per 100-mg vial

to be because of decreased uptake by the reticuloendothelial system (RES).[18] Liposomes containing amphotericin B fuse with the fungal cell membrane, leading to fungal cell death.[19] Lip-amB has been evaluated for safety in healthy beagle dogs.[20] When dogs were dosed at 1 mg/kg/d for 29 days, no azotemia was noted, and minimal renal tubular necrosis was seen on histopathology. Notably, after a single dose, peak plasma concentrations of amphotericin B that were reached after lip-amB administration were about sixfold higher than those that would be expected after comparable doses of original amphotericin B.[21] Thus, despite high plasma concentrations, lip-amB seems to spare the kidneys in dogs.

Amphotericin B lipid complex (ABLC; Abelcet, Enzon Pharmaceuticals) was the second lipid-incorporated preparation to reach the market, and is composed of a suspension of amphotericin B complexed with 2 phospholipids, dimyristoylphosphatidylcholine and dimyristoylphosphatidylglycerol, with an amphotericin B/phospholipid ratio of 1:3.[22] ABLC is taken up by the cells of the RES, and subsequently concentrates in the liver, lungs, and spleen.[23] Within ABLC, amphotericin B remains tightly bound to phospholipids, which prevents an interaction with cholesterol in mammalian membranes.[24] The lipid complexes are believed to be disrupted by phopholipases at sites of inflammation or infection, leading to the release of amphotericin B.[25] Repeated dosing of up to 5 mg/kg/d in research dogs found ABLC to be eight- to tenfold less nephrotoxic, from renal values and histology, than conventional amphotericin B deoxycholate.[26] In one report, dogs with blastomycosis were treated with ABLC at a dosage of 1 mg/kg 3 times weekly, up to a total dose of 12 mg/kg. Seven of 8 dogs receiving 12 mg/kg ABLC were considered cured, whereas 1 dog relapsed within 30 days.[27] Although mean GFR decreased during the course of treatment, only 1 of 10 dogs that received 8 to 12 mg/kg ABLC showed a decrease in GFR to less than the lower limit of the reference range.[27]

The third lipid-incorporated preparation to be developed was amphotericin B colloidal dispersion (ABCD; Amphotec, Three Rivers Pharmaceuticals). This formulation is composed of amphotericin B inserted between cholesterol sulfate bilayers, creating a disklike structure.[28] Similar to ABLC, ABCD is rapidly taken up by the RES. In one canine study, ABCD led to high concentrations in the bone marrow, liver, and spleen in healthy dogs,[29] whereas concentrations remained low in the kidneys and lungs.[14] Plasma concentrations are lower for comparable dosages of ABCD compared with conventional amphotericin B, and dosages that are nephrotoxic for the older formulation (eg, 0.6 mg/kg/d for 14 days), did not cause azotemia in dogs treated with ABCD.[30]

All 3 modified amphotericin B preparations have greater hydrophobicity, which likely results in greater delivery to the site of infection, and decreased delivery to the kidneys.[1,31] All 3 modifications seem to maintain efficacy relative to conventional amphotericin B, and decrease nephrotoxicity in humans. A meta-analysis of human studies suggests that, compared with the original formulation, the lipid amphotericin B formulations reduced all-cause mortality by 28% and the risk of doubling serum creatinine by 58%.[32] Sodium loading of human patients before amphotericin B administration seems to reduce nephrotoxicity, although the precise mechanism for this reduction remains unknown.[33,34] To increase safety, one guideline for amphotericin B use in humans includes a sodium IV bolus of 150 mEq per person along with normal dietary sodium intake.[35]

Amphotericin B has been used effectively in humans for the treatment of many systemic fungal infections, including histoplasmosis, blastomycosis, cryptococcosis, coccidioidomycosis, and aspergillosis.[36–40] The use of amphotericin B has been recommended for similar systemic fungal infections in dogs and cats.[41–45] Although the use of amphotericin B in humans has been supplanted somewhat by the development of broad-spectrum triazole drugs, such as voriconazole,[2] and echinocandins, amphotericin B remains an essential drug in human patients because of the IV route of administration and rapid onset of action.

Amphotericin B remains an important treatment option in veterinary medicine, because many of the newer drugs available for humans are cost-prohibitive in veterinary patients. Most veterinary reports describe the use of amphotericin B for life-threatening systemic mycoses, with use of the ABLC formulation reported most commonly.[27,42,45] The authors have used ABLC according to a protocol, modified from one reported previously[27] in dogs with blastomycosis, at 1 mg/kg per treatment administered every other day, up to a total dosage of 8 to 12 mg/kg (**Box 1**). This protocol is designed to provide volume expansion and diuresis, but avoid incompatibilities between lactated Ringer solution (LRS) and amphotericin B. Despite anecdotal reports of decreased nephrotoxicity associated with warming of amphotericin B before administration, no experimental or clinical studies exist to warrant this additional step.

AZOLES

Beginning with the availability of the first oral azole antifungal, ketoconazole (Nizoral, Ortho-McNeil-Janssen Pharmaceuticals), in the early 1980s, oral outpatient treatment became possible for many patients with systemic mycoses.[46,47] The azole drugs exert their effect by inhibition of lanosterol 14-α demethylase, leading to ergosterol depletion and accumulation of aberrant and potentially toxic sterols in the cell membrane.[48] Azoles are classified as imidazoles or triazoles depending on whether they possess 2 or 3 nitrogen molecules within their azole ring. Within human medicine, imidazoles have become largely reserved for topical use, whereas triazoles have become the recommended therapy for systemic disease.[49] Several azole antifungal drugs inhibit mammalian cytochrome P450 enzymes, and potential drug interactions must be

---

Box 1
Modified protocol for ABLC administration, used by the authors for the treatment of canine blastomycosis (protocol courtesy of Dr Heidi Kellihan, Madison, WI)

1 Reconstitute ABLC to a concentration of 5 mg/mL with sterile water

2 Calculate the patient's dosage (1 mg/kg) and dilute the appropriate volume of reconstituted ABLC to a concentration of 1 mg/mL in 5% dextrose in water (D5W)

3 Consider pretreatment with antiinflammatory dosages of dexamethasone (about 0.1 mg/kg IV) and metoclopramide (0.2–0.4 mg/kg IV), approximately 30 minutes before ABLC administration

4 For 30 minutes before ABLC administration, begin LRS infusion at 2.5 times the maintenance rate

5 Immediately before ABLC administration, discontinue LRS, and flush the line with D5W

6 Infuse the ABLC dose in D5W over 2 hours

7 Once the ABLC infusion is complete, flush the line with D5W

8 Restart LRS at 2.5 times the maintenance rate and continue for 120 minutes after ABLC treatment

Data from Krawiec DR, McKiernan BC, Twardock AR, et al. Use of an amphotericin B lipid complex for treatment of blastomycosis in dogs. J Am Vet Med Assoc 1996;209(12):2073–5.

considered when they are combined with other drugs.[50,51] Individual azole drugs are described later, and are summarized in **Table 2**.

Ketoconazole

Ketoconazole was the first azole released, and is the only imidazole antifungal agent remaining in use for the treatment of systemic mycoses. It is highly lipophilic, and is highly (99%) plasma protein bound in humans, which impairs distribution to the

Table 2
Summary of azole antifungal drugs, including formulation, indications, and side effects

Drug	Class and Formulation	Indications	Side Effects
Ketoconazole	Imidazole (oral, topical)	Topical mycotic infections malassezia dermatitis Third-line treatment of systemic mycoses	GI upset Dose-dependent increases in ALT Potent CYP3A inhibitor (also shown in dogs and cats) Inhibitor of p-glycoprotein Absorption impaired by antacids
Fluconazole	First-generation triazole (oral, injectable)	Candidiasis and cryptococcosis Systemic mycoses with ocular or CNS involvement Possibly first-line treatment of blastomycosis	GI upset Dose-dependent increases in ALT Requires dosage reduction in renal failure
Itraconazole	First-generation triazole (oral)	First-line for non–life-threatening systemic mycoses that do not involve CNS	GI upset Dose-dependent increases in ALT CYP3A inhibitor Absorption impaired by antacids
Voriconazole	Second-generation triazole (oral, injectable)	Invasive aspergillosis Likely efficacious against most systemic mycoses	Visual abnormalities in humans CYP3A inhibitor Induces its own metabolism over time in dogs
Posaconazole	Second-generation triazole (oral)	Aspergillosis, candidiasis, and cryptococcosis Limited data, but likely effective against other systemic mycoses	GI upset Headache Prolongation of QT interval CYP3A inhibitor
Clotrimazole	Imidazole (topical)	Sinonasal aspergillosis malassezia otitis	Poor oral bioavailability
Enilconazole	Imidazole (topical)	Sinonasal aspergillosis	Poor oral bioavailability

Abbreviations: ALT, alanine aminotransferase; CNS, central nervous system; GI, gastrointestinal.

brain and cerebrospinal fluid. Ketoconazole shows optimal dissolution and absorption at an acidic gastric pH in both humans[47] and dogs,[52] and should not be given with antacids.

For treatment of systemic mycoses, high dosages of ketoconazole (800 mg/d) are required for optimal cure rates in human patients,[53] and other, more effective azoles are recommended instead. The use of ketoconazole in humans is now largely reserved for topical administration for superficial fungal and seborrheic dermatitis.

In dogs, ketoconazole has been used historically to treat various systemic mycoses, including blastomycosis and histoplasmosis.[41,54] Although ketoconazole has been successful in treating systemic mycoses, it must be combined with amphotericin B to yield response rates that are comparable with itraconazole alone in dogs with systemic blastomycosis.[41] As in humans, triazoles such as fluconazole and itraconazole have better efficacy than ketoconazole alone,[41,44,54–56] and are the recommended treatment of both blastomycosis and histoplasmosis in dogs.[57,58] Nonetheless, ketoconazole remains an inexpensive and effective treatment of malassezia dermatitis in veterinary patients. A recent evidence-based review of malassezia dermatitis in dogs concluded that ketoconazole was effective at both 5 and 10 mg/kg per day for 3 weeks,[59] with no difference in efficacy between the lower and higher dosage. Ketoconazole is currently available as an oral tablet, or in topical cream and shampoo formulations.

Gastrointestinal upset or decreased appetite account for more than half of the adverse events reported in dogs treated with ketoconazole, with 7% of dogs exhibiting nausea or vomiting and 5% of dogs showing only inappetance[60]; similar signs are seen in treated cats.[61] Hepatotoxicity and skin reactions, including erythema and pruritus, are less frequently observed.[60] Hepatotoxicity from ketoconazole typically manifests as mild to moderate increases in alanine aminotransferase (ALT) that are reversible with drug discontinuation. More serious, but rare, reactions leading to hepatic failure have also been reported in human patients.[62] Ketoconazole hepatotoxicity has been reproduced in rodents and is dose dependent. Toxicity is caused by an oxidative metabolite, and can be ameliorated by glutathione.[63–65] However, the influence of glutathione supplementation on azole hepatotoxicity has not been evaluated in human or veterinary patients.

Ketoconazole is a potent inhibitor of both the P450 enzyme CYP3A and p-glycoprotein, and therefore has many potential drug interactions. For example, ketoconazole leads to increased plasma concentrations of ivermectin[66] and midazolam in dogs,[67] and cyclosporine in dogs and cats.[68,69] Ketoconazole inhibits the adrenal production of testosterone,[70] and should be avoided in breeding animals. In addition, because ketoconazole also inhibits cortisol synthesis,[71] the risk of adrenal suppression should be considered in treated dogs that are undergoing stressful procedures.

Fluconazole

Fluconazole (Diflucan, Pfizer) is a first-generation triazole drug that was initially released in 1990 for the treatment of candidiasis and cryptococcosis. Its in vitro susceptibility profile suggests low potency as an antifungal agent; however it is water soluble, minimally (˜10%) protein bound, and distributes well throughout the body, leading to better efficacy in vivo. Fluconazole effectively penetrates the blood-brain barrier, as well as the blood-ocular and blood-prostate barriers, in both humans and veterinary patients.[72–74] Although fluconazole may be used for the treatment of endemic systemic mycoses in humans, it does not seem to be as effective as other triazoles. Fluconazole is therefore not a first-line treatment of most systemic mycoses in humans, unless infections involve the eye or brain,[75,76] as in cryptococcal meningitis.[77] Fluconazole absorption is not affected by concurrent use of antacids,[78] and may be a better choice in patients requiring H_2-blockers or proton pump inhibitor therapy. Fluconazole also does not require food for optimal absorption.[78] Because fluconazole is excreted approximately 70% unchanged in the urine, the dosage should be reduced in patients with compromised renal function.[79,80]

As in humans, fluconazole has been recommended for veterinary patients with systemic mycoses affecting the central nervous system (CNS) or eyes. Fluconazole has been used successfully in dogs and cats with cryptococcosis and blastomycosis,[41,44,81] and the introduction of generic fluconazole has significantly reduced its cost. The investigators have routinely used fluconazole as a first-line drug for the treatment of canine systemic blastomycosis, and have found no clinically apparent difference in efficacy compared with itraconazole. In addition, the authors have switched dogs to fluconazole after the development of hepatotoxicity on itraconazole, and have found that some of these dogs tolerate fluconazole without increases in hepatic enzymes. However, we have also observed moderate ALT increases in several dogs receiving fluconazole for treatment of blastomycosis; ALT increase typically decreased or normalized following fluconazole dose reduction. Fluconazole is a teratogen in animals, and should be avoided during pregnancy.[82]

Fluconazole is empirically prescribed at a dosage of 5 to 10 mg/kg per day in dogs, whereas one feline study suggests that a dosage of 50 mg per cat per day achieves plasma concentrations that exceed minimum inhibitory concentrations for most pathogenic fungi.[74] Because of its predictable pharmacokinetics, fluconazole does not require therapeutic drug monitoring.[83] Fluconazole is available as a tablet and oral suspension, as well as an IV formulation.

Itraconazole

Itraconazole (Sporanox, Ortho-McNeil-Janssen Pharmaceuticals) is another first-generation triazole that was released shortly after fluconazole, and rapidly became the oral treatment of choice for both histoplasmosis and blastomycosis in humans. Itraconazole was also used for coccidioidomycosis, although with lower success rates.[46] Itraconazole remains the preferred azole in human patients for non–life-threatening systemic mycoses that do not involve the CNS. It is lipophilic and is highly protein bound (>99%); like ketoconazole, the absorption of itraconazole is diminished in the presence of antacids.[78,84] Therefore, it is recommended that itraconazole be administered with food, and that antacids are avoided during itraconazole therapy.

Itraconazole has become the drug of choice for treatment of systemic mycoses in dogs and cats, and is effective in the treatment of blastomycosis, histoplasmosis, cryptococcosis, and coccidioidomycosis.[41,42,55,56,85] Although itraconazole does not effectively penetrate the blood-brain or blood-ocular barriers, it may achieve levels adequate to treat CNS or ocular infection when there is associated inflammation and compromise of the barriers.

Itraconazole has been dosed at 5 to 10 mg/kg per day, and may be administered as single dose or divided into twice-daily dosing. The most common side effects are gastrointestinal upset and hepatocellular toxicity. One study found no difference in efficacy between 5 and 10 mg/kg/d in dogs treated for blastomycosis, but found a significant increase in hepatotoxicity at the higher dosage.[56] Although a loading dose of itraconazole has been suggested when starting therapy, the same study found no difference in outcome with or without an initial loading dose.[56] The investigators therefore recommended dosing itraconazole at 5 mg/kg/d for treatment of canine blastomycosis.

Substitution with generic itraconazole has been shown to reduce plasma itraconazole concentrations to the subtherapeutic range in humans, and has led to recrudescence of infection.[86] Therefore, serum itraconazole concentrations should be monitored if generic itraconazole is used and the patient does not respond promptly to therapy. Itraconazole concentrations can be measured at steady state in dogs after 2 weeks of therapy.[56] Based on human studies using high-pressure liquid chromatography measurements, plasma itraconazole concentrations should be targeted to at least 0.5 to 1.0 µg/mL.[87,88] For microbiological assays that measure both itraconazole and its active metabolite, hydroxyitraconazole, targeted concentrations should be doubled, because itraconazole and hydroxyitraconazole are present in an approximately 1:1 ratio.[89]

As with ketoconazole, itraconazole is an inhibitor of CYP3A and has many potential drug interactions. Itraconazole has been shown to increase the concentrations of cyclosporine,[90] digoxin,[91] and midazolam[92] in humans; however, these studies have not been performed in dogs or cats. Itraconazole was also found to increase methylprednisolone, but not prednisolone, concentrations in healthy humans.[93] Unlike ketoconazole, itraconazole does not seem to be a significant inhibitor of cortisol or testosterone synthesis at clinically relevant doses.[94] Itraconazole is available as an oral capsule and solution; the oral itraconazole solution has increased bioavailability compared with capsules in both humans[95] and cats.[96]

Newer Triazoles

Voriconazole (Vfend, Pfizer) is a second-generation triazole that is structurally similar to fluconazole. Voriconazole was approved in 2002, and has become the drug of choice for treatment of invasive aspergillosis in humans.[97] Despite its similarity to fluconazole, voriconazole is poorly water soluble and moderately protein bound. Studies have shown activity against *Candida* and *Aspergillus* spp as well as in vitro activity against *Blastomyces*, *Histoplasma*, *Coccidioides*, and *Cryptococcus neoformans*.[98,99]

The most common adverse effects reported in humans are blurred vision, photophobia and visual color changes, and, rarely, visual and auditory hallucinations.[100] Hepatotoxicity, skin rash or eruptions, and peripheral neuropathy have also been reported.[101–103] As for ketoconazole and itraconazole, voriconazole is a substrate inhibitor of CYP3A, and can increase plasma concentrations of other drugs in humans.[104] Voriconazole is also teratogenic in animals and should not be used during pregnancy. In dogs, voriconazole undergoes extensive metabolism; it also induces its own metabolism over time.[105] The in vitro potency of voriconazole against veterinary fungal isolates seems to be favorable compared with itraconazole.[106] Voriconazole is available as an oral tablet or solution, or as an IV preparation, but the average wholesale price for use in humans is estimated at $120/d.[4] To date, no clinical studies in veterinary patients have been reported, and its use is likely to be cost-prohibitive in the near future.

Posaconazole (Noxafil, Schering-Plough) is a lipophilic second-generation triazole derived from itraconazole. Posaconazole was approved in 2006 for prophylaxis of invasive *Aspergillus* and *Candida* infections and for treatment of oropharyngeal candidiasis.[4] It shows excellent in vitro activity against these organisms, as well as *C neoformans*.[107,108] Posaconazole also seems to have efficacy against *Blastomyces*, *Histoplasma*, and *Coccidioides* spp, but clinical use and experience remains limited even in human patients.[109,110] As with itraconazole, administration of posaconazole with a meal (especially high in fat) seems to improve bioavailability; however, like fluconazole, alterations in gastric acidity do not seem to affect posaconazole absorption.[111,112]

The most common adverse effects reported in human patients are headache and gastrointestinal upset; hepatotoxicity and QT interval prolongation are much less common.[113] Although posaconazole seems to have a narrower drug interaction profile, inhibition of CYP3A4 has been shown in humans.[114] This interaction has been shown to increase serum concentrations of tacrolimus and cyclosporine.[115] No IV formulations are available, and a recent review[4] reported the average wholesale price of posaconazole for use in humans to be $115/d. As with voriconazole, the use of posaconazole is likely to be restricted in veterinary patients until an effective generic formulation is available.

Topical Azoles

Both clotrimazole (Taro Pharmaceuticals) and enilconazole (Merial) are classified as imidazoles within the azole class of drugs; however, both drugs have minimal systemic bioavailability because of a high first-pass effect; this finding has also been shown with clotrimazole in dogs.[116] These drugs are therefore confined to topical use, such as clotrimazole in otic suspensions for the treatment of malassezia otitis in dogs and cats.[117] Both clotrimazole and enilconazole are effective, when instilled into the nasal passages, for treating sinonasal aspergillosis in dogs[118,119]; clotrimazole has also been reported to be effective in cats with nasal aspergillosis.[120,121] The comparative efficacy and long-term outcomes of enilconazole versus clotrimazole for sinonasal aspergillosis have not been evaluated. One-hour infusions of 1% clotrimazole solution or 1% to 2% enilconazole solution, combined with appropriate debridement of fungal plaques, seem to be effective in curing approximately 50% to 65% of dogs with a single treatment.[122–124] Although some dogs require multiple treatments, more than 85% of dogs can be cured with up to 3 treatments.[122,123] Side effects are uncommon, although 1 dog treated with clotrimazole reportedly developed severe pharyngitis and upper airway edema.[125] However, this reaction was proposed to be secondary to the propylene glycol and isopropyl alcohol used as the carriers, rather than the clotrimazole itself. A veterinary product containing 1% clotrimazole solution (Vétoquinol USA) is available; however, this product contains propylene glycol. Therefore, the authors recommend using human clotrimazole products for intranasal infusion; these are formulated in polyethylene glycol, which has not been associated with pharyngitis.

ECHINOCANDINS

Echinocandins are a fairly new class of antifungal medications; the first compound, caspofungin (Cancidas, Merck) was approved by the US Food and Drug Administration in 2001. Echinocandins inhibit glucan synthase and prevent the synthesis of β-1,3 glucan, an essential component of the cell wall in certain fungi.[2,126,127] In susceptible fungi, the integrity of the cell wall is compromised, leading to cell lysis.[128] A second mechanism of action may be through disruption of cell wall mannoproteins, which leads to greater exposed antigen and subsequently greater immune system recognition.[129]

The clinical use of the echinocandins is limited to Candida and Aspergillus spp in human patients; C neoformans and the zygomycetes (opportunistic infectious agents including Rhizopus spp) are typically resistant.[127,130] The mycelial forms of Blastomyces dermatitidis and Histoplasma capsulatum seem to be susceptible to the echinocandins, although the yeast forms are not, because of the predominance of α-glucan, which is not a target of echinocandins, in the yeast cell wall.[131] Echinocandins have poor oral bioavailability and are only available in IV formulations.[127,132] The side effects associated with echinocandins are typically minimal, with fever, gastrointestinal signs, phlebitis, and headache being most commonly reported.[133–135]

Caspofungin is approved for salvage therapy in patients with invasive aspergillosis. In addition to caspofungin, micafungin (Mycamine, Astellas Pharma) and anidulafungin (Eraxis, Pfizer) are also approved for treatment of candidemia and esophageal candidiasis.[127] Although these drugs may hold promise for the treatment of systemic aspergillosis in veterinary patients, their potential to treat the common dimorphic fungal infections in dogs and cats is poor because of their lack of efficacy against the yeast forms of fungi.

TERBINAFINE

Terbinafine (Lamisil, Novartis) belongs to the allylamine group of antifungal agents, and is most frequently used in humans for the treatment of dermatophytoses and toenail onychomycosis.[136,137] Its antifungal activity is mediated via noncompetitive inhibition of squalene epoxidase, an enzyme involved in fungal ergosterol synthesis, with more than 4000-fold selectivity for fungal versus mammalian P450 enzymes.[138] The pharmacokinetics of terbinafine differ substantially from other antifungal agents; this drug is well absorbed from the gastrointestinal tract and then rapidly diffuses from the bloodstream into the dermis and epidermis. Terbinafine is highly lipophilic, which leads to its high concentration in hair follicles, skin, nail plate, and adipose tissue, with levels in the stratum corneum exceeding those in plasma by a factor of 75 within 12 days of therapy.[139,140]

Terbinafine has shown high in vitro efficacy against many dermatophytes, including *Trichophyton* and *Tinea* spp, and has largely replaced the use of griseofulvin for the management of most dermatomycoses and ringworm infections in humans.[136,140,141] Terbinafine has also been combined with echinocandins or triazoles in a multimodal approach to systemic mycoses in humans.[136] Side effects are generally limited to gastrointestinal upset and, rarely, hepatotoxicity.[140] Terbinafine is currently available in tablet form as well as a topical cream or gel.

In dogs, terbinafine has in vitro activity against *Microsporum* and *Trichophyton* isolates, with little evidence of acquired resistance during treatment.[142] Terbinafine seems to be equivalent or superior to ketoconazole for the treatment of malassezia dermatitis in dogs, with a reduction in both yeast counts and pruritus.[143,144]

SUMMARY

Although the number of antifungal agents available in the marketplace is increasing, the options for treating veterinary patients with systemic mycoses remain limited. Non–life-threatening or non-CNS infections resulting from *B dermatitidis*, *H capsulatum*, and *Coccidioides immitis* can initially be treated with either fluconazole or itraconazole, although there is more experience with itraconazole. In cases of CNS or ocular involvement, or *C neoformans* infection, fluconazole may be considered the preferred treatment; it is also considerably less expensive than itraconazole. If a systemic fungal infection is considered life threatening, or if a patient is diagnosed with systemic aspergillosis, amphotericin B therapy may be indicated because of its rapid onset of action and greater efficacy against *Aspergillus* spp. The use of ketoconazole and terbinafine is largely reserved for topical fungal infections. In the future, newer triazoles and echinocandins may become more affordable and expand the options available to veterinary patients.

REFERENCES

1. Saliba F, Dupont B. Renal impairment and amphotericin B formulations in patients with invasive fungal infections. Med Mycol 2008;46(2):97–112.
2. Thompson GR 3rd, Cadena J, Patterson TF. Overview of antifungal agents. Clin Chest Med 2009;30(2):203–15, v.
3. Spanakis EK, Aperis G, Mylonakis E. New agents for the treatment of fungal infections: clinical efficacy and gaps in coverage. Clin Infect Dis 2006;43(8):1060–8.
4. Rachwalski EJ, Wieczorkiewicz JT, Scheetz MH. Posaconazole: an oral triazole with an extended spectrum of activity. Ann Pharmacother 2008;42(10):1429–38.
5. Brajtburg J, Bolard J. Carrier effects on biological activity of amphotericin B. Clin Microbiol Rev 1996;9(4):512–31.
6. Bolard J. How do the polyene macrolide antibiotics affect the cellular membrane properties? Biochim Biophys Acta 1986;864(3-4):257–304.
7. Gallis HA, Drew RH, Pickard WW. Amphotericin B: 30 years of clinical experience. Rev Infect Dis 1990;12(2):308–29.
8. Khoo SH, Bond J, Denning DW. Administering amphotericin B–a practical approach. J Antimicrob Chemother 1994;33(2):203–13.
9. Costa S, Nucci M. Can we decrease amphotericin nephrotoxicity? Curr Opin Crit Care 2001;7(6):379–83.
10. Gerkens JF, Branch RA. The influence of sodium status and furosemide on canine acute amphotericin B nephrotoxicity. J Pharmacol Exp Ther 1980; 214(2):306–11.
11. Sawaya BP, Weihprecht H, Campbell WR, et al. Direct vasoconstriction as a possible cause for amphotericin B-induced nephrotoxicity in rats. J Clin Invest 1991;87(6):2097–107.
12. Ohnishi A, Ohnishi T, Stevenhead W, et al. Sodium status influences chronic amphotericin B nephrotoxicity in rats. Antimicrobial Agents Chemother 1989;33(8): 1222–7.
13. Walsh TJ, Hiemenz JW, Seibel NL, et al. Amphotericin B lipid complex for invasive fungal infections: analysis of safety and efficacy in 556 cases. Clin Infect Dis 1998;26(6):1383–96.
14. Herbrecht R, Natarajan-Ame S, Nivoix Y, et al. The lipid formulations of amphotericin B. Expert Opin Pharmacother 2003;4(8):1277–87.
15. Hiemenz JW, Walsh TJ. Lipid formulations of amphotericin B: recent progress and future directions. Clin Infect Dis 1996;22(Suppl 2):S133–44.
16. Tiphine M, Letscher-Bru V, Herbrecht R. Amphotericin B and its new formulations: pharmacologic characteristics, clinical efficacy, and tolerability. Transpl Infect Dis 1999;1(4):273–83.
17. Hay RJ. Liposomal amphotericin B, AmBisome. J Infect 1994;28(Suppl 1): 35–43.
18. de Marie S, Janknegt R, Bakker-Woudenberg IA. Clinical use of liposomal and lipid–complexed amphotericin B. J Antimicrob Chemother 1994;33(5):907–16.
19. Adler-Moore J. AmBisome targeting to fungal infections. Bone Marrow Transplant 1994;14(Suppl 5):S3–7.
20. Bekersky I, Boswell GW, Hiles R, et al. Safety and toxicokinetics of intravenous liposomal amphotericin B (AmBisome) in beagle dogs. Pharm Res 1999;16(11): 1694–701.
21. Kim H, Loebenberg D, Marco A, et al. Comparative pharmacokinetics of SCH 28191 and amphotericin B in mice, rats, dogs, and cynomolgus monkeys. Antimicrobial Agents Chemother 1984;26(4):446–9.

22. Janoff AS, Boni LT, Popescu MC, et al. Unusual lipid structures selectively reduce the toxicity of amphotericin B. Proc Natl Acad Sci U S A 1988;85(16): 6122–6.
23. Olsen SJ, Swerdel MR, Blue B, et al. Tissue distribution of amphotericin B lipid complex in laboratory animals. J Pharm Pharmacol 1991;43(12):831–5.
24. Adedoyin A, Swenson CE, Bolcsak LE, et al. A pharmacokinetic study of amphotericin B lipid complex injection (Abelcet) in patients with definite or probable systemic fungal infections. Antimicrobial Agents Chemother 2000;44(10):2900–2.
25. Swenson CE, Perkins WR, Roberts P, et al. In vitro and in vivo antifungal activity of amphotericin B lipid complex: are phospholipases important? Antimicrobial Agents Chemother 1998;42(4):767–71.
26. Janoff AS, Perkins WR, Saletan SL, et al. Amphotericin B lipid complex (ABLC™):a molecular rationale for the attenuation of amphotericin B related toxicities. J Liposome Res 1993;3(3):451–71.
27. Krawiec DR, McKiernan BC, Twardock AR, et al. Use of an amphotericin B lipid complex for treatment of blastomycosis in dogs. J Am Vet Med Assoc 1996; 209(12):2073–5.
28. de Marie S. Liposomal and lipid-based formulations of amphotericin B. Leukemia 1996;10(Suppl 2):s93–6.
29. Herbrecht R, Letscher V, Andres E, et al. Safety and efficacy of amphotericin B colloidal dispersion. An overview. Chemotherapy 1999;45(Suppl 1):67–76.
30. Fielding RM, Singer AW, Wang LH, et al. Relationship of pharmacokinetics and drug distribution in tissue to increased safety of amphotericin B colloidal dispersion in dogs. Antimicrobial Agents Chemother 1992;36(2):299–307.
31. Wong-Beringer A, Jacobs RA, Guglielmo BJ. Lipid formulations of amphotericin B: clinical efficacy and toxicities. Clin Infect Dis 1998;27(3):603–18.
32. Barrett JP, Vardulaki KA, Conlon C, et al. A systematic review of the antifungal effectiveness and tolerability of amphotericin B formulations. Clin Ther 2003; 25(5):1295–320.
33. Llanos A, Cieza J, Bernardo J, et al. Effect of salt supplementation on amphotericin B nephrotoxicity. Kidney Int 1991;40(2):302–8.
34. Turcu R, Patterson MJ, Omar S. Influence of sodium intake on amphotericin B-induced nephrotoxicity among extremely premature infants. Pediatr Nephrol 2009;24(3):497–505.
35. Anderson CM. Sodium chloride treatment of amphotericin B nephrotoxicity. Standard of care? West J Med 1995;162(4):313–7.
36. Del Bono V, Mikulska M, Viscoli C. Invasive aspergillosis: diagnosis, prophylaxis and treatment. Curr Opin Hematol 2008;15(6):586–93.
37. Knoper SR, Galgiani JN. Systemic fungal infections: diagnosis and treatment. I. Coccidioidomycosis. Infect Dis Clin North Am 1988;2(4):861–75.
38. Kotwani RN, Gokhale PC, Bodhe PV, et al. Safety and efficacy of liposomal amphotericin B in patients with cryptococcal meningitis. J Assoc Physicians India 2001;49:1086–90.
39. Saag MS, Dismukes WE. Treatment of histoplasmosis and blastomycosis. Chest 1988;93(4):848–51.
40. Taylor RL, Williams DM, Craven PC, et al. Amphotericin B in liposomes: a novel therapy for histoplasmosis. Am Rev Respir Dis 1982;125(5):610–1.
41. Arceneaux KA, Taboada J, Hosgood G. Blastomycosis in dogs: 115 cases (1980–1995). J Am Vet Med Assoc 1998;213(5):658–64.
42. Graupmann-Kuzma A, Valentine BA, Shubitz LF, et al. Coccidioidomycosis in dogs and cats: a review. J Am Anim Hosp Assoc 2008;44(5):226–35.

43. Mitchell M, Stark DR. Disseminated canine histoplasmosis: a clinical survey of 24 cases in Texas. Can Vet J 1980;21(3):95–100.

44. O'Brien CR, Krockenberger MB, Martin P, et al. Long-term outcome of therapy for 59 cats and 11 dogs with cryptococcosis. Aust Vet J 2006; 84(11):384–92.

45. Schultz RM, Johnson EG, Wisner ER, et al. Clinicopathologic and diagnostic imaging characteristics of systemic aspergillosis in 30 dogs. J Vet Intern Med 2008;22(4):851–9.

46. Kauffman CA. Role of azoles in antifungal therapy. Clin Infect Dis 1996;22(Suppl 2): S148–53.

47. Sheehan DJ, Hitchcock CA, Sibley CM. Current and emerging azole antifungal agents. Clin Microbiol Rev 1999;12(1):40–79.

48. Groll AH, De Lucca AJ, Walsh TJ. Emerging targets for the development of novel antifungal therapeutics. Trends Microbiol 1998;6(3):117–24.

49. Zonios DI, Bennett JE. Update on azole antifungals. Semin Respir Crit Care Med 2008;29(2):198–210.

50. Como JA, Dismukes WE. Oral azole drugs as systemic antifungal therapy. N Engl J Med 1994;330(4):263–72.

51. Pea F, Furlanut M. Pharmacokinetic aspects of treating infections in the intensive care unit: focus on drug interactions. Clin Pharmacokinet 2001;40(11):833–68.

52. Zhou R, Moench P, Heran C, et al. pH-dependent dissolution in vitro and absorption in vivo of weakly basic drugs: development of a canine model. Pharm Res 2005;22(2):188–92.

53. Treatment of blastomycosis and histoplasmosis with ketoconazole. Results of a prospective randomized clinical trial. National institute of allergy and infectious diseases mycoses study group. Ann Intern Med 1985;103(6 (Pt 1)): 861–72.

54. Clinkenbeard KD, Cowell RL, Tyler RD. Disseminated histoplasmosis in dogs: 12 cases (1981–1986). J Am Vet Med Assoc 1988;193(11):1443–7.

55. Hodges RD, Legendre AM, Adams LG, et al. Itraconazole for the treatment of histoplasmosis in cats. J Vet Intern Med 1994;8(6):409–13.

56. Legendre AM, Rohrbach BW, Toal RL, et al. Treatment of blastomycosis with itraconazole in 112 dogs. J Vet Intern Med 1996;10(6):365–71.

57. Bromel C, Sykes JE. Epidemiology, diagnosis, and treatment of blastomycosis in dogs and cats. Clin Tech Small Anim Pract 2005;20(4):233–9.

58. Bromel C, Sykes JE. Histoplasmosis in dogs and cats. Clin Tech Small Anim Pract 2005;20(4):227–32.

59. Negre A, Bensignor E, Guillot J. Evidence-based veterinary dermatology: a systematic review of interventions for malassezia dermatitis in dogs. Vet Dermatol 2009;20(1):1–12.

60. Mayer UK, Glos K, Schmid M, et al. Adverse effects of ketoconazole in dogs– a retrospective study. Vet Dermatol 2008;19(4):199–208.

61. Medleau L, Chalmers SA. Ketoconazole for treatment of dermatophytosis in cats. J Am Vet Med Assoc 1992;200(1):77–8.

62. Brusko CS, Marten JT. Ketoconazole hepatotoxicity in a patient treated for environmental illness and systemic candidiasis. DICP 1991;25(12):1321–5.

63. Rodriguez RJ, Acosta D Jr. Comparison of ketoconazole- and fluconazole-induced hepatotoxicity in a primary culture system of rat hepatocytes. Toxicology 1995;96(2):83–92.

64. Rodriguez RJ, Acosta D Jr. N-deacetyl ketoconazole-induced hepatotoxicity in a primary culture system of rat hepatocytes. Toxicology 1997;117(2-3):123–31.

65. Rodriguez RJ, Buckholz CJ. Hepatotoxicity of ketoconazole in Sprague-Dawley rats: glutathione depletion, flavin-containing monooxygenases-mediated bioactivation and hepatic covalent binding. Xenobiotica 2003;33(4):429–41.

66. Hugnet C, Lespine A, Alvinerie M. Multiple oral dosing of ketoconazole increases dog exposure to ivermectin. J Pharm Pharm Sci 2007;10(3):311–8.

67. Kuroha M, Azumano A, Kuze Y, et al. Effect of multiple dosing of ketoconazole on pharmacokinetics of midazolam, a cytochrome P-450 3A substrate in beagle dogs. Drug Metab Dispos 2002;30(1):63–8.

68. Dahlinger J, Gregory C, Bea J. Effect of ketoconazole on cyclosporine dose in healthy dogs. Vet Surg 1998;27(1):64–8.

69. McAnulty JF, Lensmeyer GL. The effects of ketoconazole on the pharmacokinetics of cyclosporine A in cats. Vet Surg 1999;28(6):448–55.

70. De Coster R, Beerens D, Dom J, et al. Endocrinological effects of single daily ketoconazole administration in male beagle dogs. Acta Endocrinol (Copenh) 1984;107(2):275–81.

71. Lien YH, Huang HP. Use of ketoconazole to treat dogs with pituitary-dependent hyperadrenocorticism: 48 cases (1994–2007). J Am Vet Med Assoc 2008;233(12):1896–901.

72. Brammer KW, Farrow PR, Faulkner JK. Pharmacokinetics and tissue penetration of fluconazole in humans. Rev Infect Dis 1990;12(Suppl 3):S318–26.

73. Latimer FG, Colitz CM, Campbell NB, et al. Pharmacokinetics of fluconazole following intravenous and oral administration and body fluid concentrations of fluconazole following repeated oral dosing in horses. Am J Vet Res 2001;62(10):1606–11.

74. Vaden SL, Heit MC, Hawkins EC, et al. Fluconazole in cats: pharmacokinetics following intravenous and oral administration and penetration into cerebrospinal fluid, aqueous humour and pulmonary epithelial lining fluid. J Vet Pharmacol Ther 1997;20(3):181–6.

75. Diaz M, Negroni R, Montero-Gei F, et al. A pan-American 5-year study of fluconazole therapy for deep mycoses in the immunocompetent host. Pan-American Study Group. Clin Infect Dis 1992;14(Suppl 1):S68–76.

76. Pappas PG, Bradsher RW, Chapman SW, et al. Treatment of blastomycosis with fluconazole: a pilot study. The National Institute of Allergy and Infectious Diseases Mycoses Study Group. Clin Infect Dis 1995;20(2):267–71.

77. Saag MS, Powderly WG, Cloud GA, et al. Comparison of amphotericin B with fluconazole in the treatment of acute AIDS-associated cryptococcal meningitis. The NIAID mycoses study group and the AIDS clinical trials group. N Engl J Med 1992;326(2):83–9.

78. Lim SG, Sawyerr AM, Hudson M, et al. Short report: the absorption of fluconazole and itraconazole under conditions of low intragastric acidity. Aliment Pharmacol Ther 1993;7(3):317–21.

79. Humphrey MJ, Jevons S, Tarbit MH. Pharmacokinetic evaluation of UK-49,858, a metabolically stable triazole antifungal drug, in animals and humans. Antimicrobial Agents Chemother 1985;28(5):648–53.

80. Jezequel SG. Fluconazole: interspecies scaling and allometric relationships of pharmacokinetic properties. J Pharm Pharmacol 1994;46(3):196–9.

81. Malik R, Wigney DI, Muir DB, et al. Cryptococcosis in cats: clinical and mycological assessment of 29 cases and evaluation of treatment using orally administered fluconazole. J Med Vet Mycol 1992;30(2):133–44.

82. Pursley TJ, Blomquist IK, Abraham J, et al. Fluconazole-induced congenital anomalies in three infants. Clin Infect Dis 1996;22(2):336–40.

83. Smith J, Andes D. Therapeutic drug monitoring of antifungals: pharmacokinetic and pharmacodynamic considerations. Ther Drug Monit 2008;30(2):167–72.

84. Kanda Y, Kami M, Matsuyama T, et al. Plasma concentration of itraconazole in patients receiving chemotherapy for hematological malignancies: the effect of famotidine on the absorption of itraconazole. Hematol Oncol 1998;16(1): 33–7.

85. Jacobs GJ, Medleau L, Calvert C, et al. Cryptococcal infection in cats: factors influencing treatment outcome, and results of sequential serum antigen titers in 35 cats. J Vet Intern Med 1997;11(1):1–4.

86. Pasqualotto AC, Denning DW. Generic substitution of itraconazole resulting in sub-therapeutic levels and resistance. Int J Antimicrob Agents 2007;30(1):93–4.

87. Denning DW, Tucker RM, Hanson LH, et al. Itraconazole therapy for crypto-coccal meningitis and cryptococcosis. Arch Intern Med 1989;149(10):2301–8.

88. Glasmacher A, Hahn C, Leutner C, et al. Breakthrough invasive fungal infections in neutropenic patients after prophylaxis with itraconazole. Mycoses 1999; 42(7–8):443–51.

89. Warnock DW, Turner A, Burke J. Comparison of high performance liquid chro-matographic and microbiological methods for determination of itraconazole. J Antimicrob Chemother 1988;21(1):93–100.

90. Kramer MR, Marshall SE, Denning DW, et al. Cyclosporine and itraconazole interaction in heart and lung transplant recipients. Ann Intern Med 1990; 113(4):327–9.

91. Sachs MK, Blanchard LM, Green PJ. Interaction of itraconazole and digoxin. Clin Infect Dis 1993;16(3):400–3.

92. Olkkola KT, Backman JT, Neuvonen PJ. Midazolam should be avoided in patients receiving the systemic antimycotics ketoconazole or itraconazole. Clin Pharmacol Ther 1994;55(5):481–5.

93. Lebrun-Vignes B, Archer VC, Diquet B, et al. Effect of itraconazole on the phar-macokinetics of prednisolone and methylprednisolone and cortisol secretion in healthy subjects. Br J Clin Pharmacol 2001;51(5):443–50.

94. Haria M, Bryson HM, Goa KL. Itraconazole. A reappraisal of its pharmacological properties and therapeutic use in the management of superficial fungal infec-tions. Drugs 1996;51(4):585–620.

95. Barone JA, Moskovitz BL, Guarnieri J, et al. Enhanced bioavailability of itraco-nazole in hydroxypropyl-beta-cyclodextrin solution versus capsules in healthy volunteers. Antimicrobial Agents Chemother 1998;42(7):1862–5.

96. Boothe DM, Herring I, Calvin J, et al. Itraconazole disposition after single oral and intravenous and multiple oral dosing in healthy cats. Am J Vet Res 1997; 58(8):872–7.

97. Herbrecht R, Denning DW, Patterson TF, et al. Voriconazole versus amphotericin B for primary therapy of invasive aspergillosis. N Engl J Med 2002;347(6): 408–15.

98. Johnson LB, Kauffman CA. Voriconazole: a new triazole antifungal agent. Clin Infect Dis 2003;36(5):630–7.

99. Li RK, Ciblak MA, Nordoff N, et al. In vitro activities of voriconazole, itraconazole, and amphotericin B against *Blastomyces dermatitidis*, *Coccidioides immitis*, and *Histoplasma capsulatum*. Antimicrobial Agents Chemother 2000;44(6): 1734–6.

100. Walsh TJ, Pappas P, Winston DJ, et al. Voriconazole compared with liposomal amphotericin B for empirical antifungal therapy in patients with neutropenia and persistent fever. N Engl J Med 2002;346(4):225–34.

101. Scherpbier HJ, Hilhorst MI, Kuijpers TW. Liver failure in a child receiving highly active antiretroviral therapy and voriconazole. Clin Infect Dis 2003; 37(6):828–30.

102. Tsiodras S, Zafiropoulou R, Kanta E, et al. Painful peripheral neuropathy associated with voriconazole use. Arch Neurol 2005;62(1):144–6.

103. Vandecasteele SJ, Van Wijngaerden E, Peetermans WE. Two cases of severe phototoxic reactions related to long-term outpatient treatment with voriconazole. Eur J Clin Microbiol Infect Dis 2004;23(8):656–7.

104. Cronin S, Chandrasekar PH. Safety of triazole antifungal drugs in patients with cancer. J Antimicrob Chemother 2010;65(3):410–6.

105. Roffey SJ, Cole S, Comby P, et al. The disposition of voriconazole in mouse, rat, rabbit, guinea pig, dog, and human. Drug Metab Dispos 2003;31(6):731–41.

106. Okabayashi K, Imaji M, Osumi T, et al. Antifungal activity of itraconazole and voriconazole against clinical isolates obtained from animals with mycoses. Nippon Ishinkin Gakkai Zasshi 2009;50(2):91–4.

107. Diekema DJ, Messer SA, Hollis RJ, et al. Activities of caspofungin, itraconazole, posaconazole, ravuconazole, voriconazole, and amphotericin B against 448 recent clinical isolates of filamentous fungi. J Clin Microbiol 2003;41(8):3623–6.

108. Pfaller MA, Messer SA, Boyken L, et al. Global trends in the antifungal susceptibility of Cryptococcus neoformans (1990 to 2004). J Clin Microbiol 2005;43(5): 2163–7.

109. Catanzaro A, Cloud GA, Stevens DA, et al. Safety, tolerance, and efficacy of posaconazole therapy in patients with nonmeningeal disseminated or chronic pulmonary coccidioidomycosis. Clin Infect Dis 2007;45(5):562–8.

110. Espinel-Ingroff A. Comparison of in vitro activities of the new triazole SCH56592 and the echinocandins MK-0991 (L-743,872) and LY303366 against opportunistic filamentous and dimorphic fungi and yeasts. J Clin Microbiol 1998; 36(10):2950–6.

111. Courtney R, Radwanski E, Lim J, et al. Pharmacokinetics of posaconazole coadministered with antacid in fasting or nonfasting healthy men. Antimicrobial Agents Chemother 2004;48(3):804–8.

112. Courtney R, Wexler D, Radwanski E, et al. Effect of food on the relative bioavailability of two oral formulations of posaconazole in healthy adults. Br J Clin Pharmacol 2004;57(2):218–22.

113. Cornely OA, Maertens J, Winston DJ, et al. Posaconazole vs. fluconazole or itraconazole prophylaxis in patients with neutropenia. N Engl J Med 2007;356(4): 348–59.

114. Wexler D, Courtney R, Richards W, et al. Effect of posaconazole on cytochrome P450 enzymes: a randomized, open-label, two-way crossover study. Eur J Pharm Sci 2004;21(5):645–53.

115. Sansone-Parsons A, Krishna G, Martinho M, et al. Effect of oral posaconazole on the pharmacokinetics of cyclosporine and tacrolimus. Pharmacotherapy 2007; 27(6):825–34.

116. Conte L, Ramis J, Mis R, et al. Pharmacokinetic study of [14C]flutrimazole after oral and intravenous administration in dogs. Comparison with clotrimazole. Arzneimittelforschung 1992;42(6):854–8.

117. Bensignor E, Grandemange E. Comparison of an antifungal agent with a mixture of antifungal, antibiotic and corticosteroid agents for the treatment of Malassezia species otitis in dogs. Vet Rec 2006;158(6):193–5.

118. Benitah N. Canine nasal aspergillosis. Clin Tech Small Anim Pract 2006;21(2): 82–8.

119. Peeters D, Clercx C. Update on canine sinonasal aspergillosis. Vet Clin North Am Small Anim Pract 2007;37(5):901–16, vi.
120. Furrow E, Groman RP. Intranasal infusion of clotrimazole for the treatment of nasal aspergillosis in two cats. J Am Vet Med Assoc 2009;235(10):1188–93.
121. Tomsa K, Glaus TM, Zimmer C, et al. Fungal rhinitis and sinusitis in three cats. J Am Vet Med Assoc 2003;222(10):1380–4, 1365.
122. Mathews KG, Davidson AP, Koblik PD, et al. Comparison of topical administration of clotrimazole through surgically placed versus nonsurgically placed catheters for treatment of nasal aspergillosis in dogs: 60 cases (1990-1996). J Am Vet Med Assoc 1998;213(4):501–6.
123. Schuller S, Clercx C. Long-term outcomes in dogs with sinonasal aspergillosis treated with intranasal infusions of enilconazole. J Am Anim Hosp Assoc 2007;43(1):33–8.
124. Zonderland JL, Stork CK, Saunders JH, et al. Intranasal infusion of enilconazole for treatment of sinonasal aspergillosis in dogs. J Am Vet Med Assoc 2002; 221(10):1421–5.
125. Caulkett N, Lew L, Fries C. Upper-airway obstruction and prolonged recovery from anesthesia following intranasal clotrimazole administration. J Am Anim Hosp Assoc 1997;33(3):264–7.
126. Sucher AJ, Chahine EB, Balcer HE. Echinocandins: the newest class of antifungals. Ann Pharmacother 2009;43(10):1647–57.
127. Turner MS, Drew RH, Perfect JR. Emerging echinocandins for treatment of invasive fungal infections. Expert Opin Emerg Drugs 2006;11(2):231–50.
128. Cappelletty D, Eiselstein-McKitrick K. The echinocandins. Pharmacotherapy 2007;27(3):369–88.
129. Lamaris GA, Lewis RE, Chamilos G, et al. Caspofungin-mediated beta-glucan unmasking and enhancement of human polymorphonuclear neutrophil activity against Aspergillus and non-Aspergillus hyphae. J Infect Dis 2008;198(2): 186–92.
130. Tawara S, Ikeda F, Maki K, et al. In vitro activities of a new lipopeptide antifungal agent, FK463, against a variety of clinically important fungi. Antimicrobial Agents Chemother 2000;44(1):57–62.
131. Nakai T, Uno J, Ikeda F, et al. In vitro antifungal activity of Micafungin (FK463) against dimorphic fungi: comparison of yeast-like and mycelial forms. Antimicrobial Agents Chemother 2003;47(4):1376–81.
132. Chandrasekar PH, Sobel JD. Micafungin: a new echinocandin. Clin Infect Dis 2006;42(8):1171–8.
133. Krause DS, Reinhardt J, Vazquez JA, et al. Phase 2, randomized, dose-ranging study evaluating the safety and efficacy of anidulafungin in invasive candidiasis and candidemia. Antimicrobial Agents Chemother 2004;48(6):2021–4.
134. van Burik JA, Ratanatharathorn V, Stepan DE, et al. Micafungin versus fluconazole for prophylaxis against invasive fungal infections during neutropenia in patients undergoing hematopoietic stem cell transplantation. Clin Infect Dis 2004;39(10):1407–16.
135. Villanueva A, Gotuzzo E, Arathoon EG, et al. A randomized double-blind study of caspofungin versus fluconazole for the treatment of esophageal candidiasis. Am J Med 2002;113(4):294–9.
136. Krishnan-Natesan S. Terbinafine: a pharmacological and clinical review. Expert Opin Pharmacother 2009;10(16):2723–33.
137. Shear NH, Villars VV, Marsolais C. Terbinafine: an oral and topical antifungal agent. Clin Dermatol 1991;9(4):487–95.

138. Ryder NS. Terbinafine: mode of action and properties of the squalene epoxidase inhibition. Br J Dermatol 1992;126(Suppl 39):2–7.

139. Faergemann J, Zehender H, Denouel J, et al. Levels of terbinafine in plasma, stratum corneum, dermis-epidermis (without stratum corneum), sebum, hair and nails during and after 250 mg terbinafine orally once per day for four weeks. Acta Derm Venereol 1993;73(4):305–9.

140. McClellan KJ, Wiseman LR, Markham A. Terbinafine. An update of its use in superficial mycoses. Drugs 1999;58(1):179–202.

141. Gupta AK, Cooper EA. Update in antifungal therapy of dermatophytosis. Mycopathologia 2008;166(5–6):353–67.

142. Hofbauer B, Leitner I, Ryder NS. In vitro susceptibility of *Microsporum canis* and other dermatophyte isolates from veterinary infections during therapy with terbinafine or griseofulvin. Med Mycol 2002;40(2):179–83.

143. Guillot J, Bensignor E, Jankowski F, et al. Comparative efficacies of oral ketoconazole and terbinafine for reducing *Malassezia* population sizes on the skin of Basset Hounds. Vet Dermatol 2003;14(3):153–7.

144. Rosales MS, Marsella R, Kunkle G, et al. Comparison of the clinical efficacy of oral terbinafine and ketoconazole combined with cephalexin in the treatment of *Malassezia* dermatitis in dogs–a pilot study. Vet Dermatol 2005;16(3):171–6.

Molecular Diagnostic Assays for Infectious Diseases in Cats

Julia K. Veir, DVM, PhD*, Michael R. Lappin, DVM, PhD

KEYWORDS

- Feline • Polymerase chain reaction • Infectious disease
- Real-time polymerase chain reaction • Diagnosis

Numerous options are available for the diagnosis of infectious diseases in feline medicine. Historically, cytologic techniques, histopathologic techniques, and microbiological cultures are used for the demonstration of the presence of the organism and serologic antibody titers for the demonstration of immune response to an infection. However, these techniques have inherent deficiencies. Cytologic and histopathologic techniques require the organism to be large enough to be seen microscopically and in sufficient numbers for visualization. The sensitivity of organism visualization for diagnosis often decreases as disease progresses because the host's immune response decreases the number of organisms in the body. Microbiological culture requires specific knowledge of the organism's requirements for growth and may require specific handling for organism preservation and culture periods longer than are clinically useful. Immune response to an organism, as demonstrated by serum antibody titers, can be sensitive but requires days to weeks for a host response and demonstrates only exposure to the organism and not the disease secondary to the organism or even the current infection.

For a diagnostic test to be practical, it must be useful (high sensitivity and specificity), reliable (reproducibility), convenient, and cost-effective. For these reasons, the use of molecular assays in feline medicine has gained favor for the diagnosis of diseases caused by organisms that are difficult to be identified, detected, or cultured in a timely fashion. Because most veterinarians rely on the proper use of molecular assays on a daily basis to practice high-quality veterinary medicine, this article provides a brief overview of the technologies available, their shortcomings and advantages, and the current clinical applications of the technologies in feline medicine.

Molecular assays rely on the detection of the nucleic acids DNA and RNA. These nucleic acids are a part of the genetic makeup of the organism and consist

Department of Clinical Sciences, Colorado State University, Campus Delivery 1620, Fort Collins, CO 80523, USA
* Corresponding author.
E-mail address: jveir@colostate.edu

Vet Clin Small Anim 40 (2010) 1189–1200
doi:10.1016/j.cvsm.2010.07.012
0195-5616/10/$ – see front matter © 2010 Elsevier Inc. All rights reserved.

vetsmall.theclinics.com

of 4 nucleotides in varying sequences. Many portions of DNA and RNA are highly conserved between organisms, whereas other portions are specific to the organism on a family, genus, species, or even strain level. The sequence specificity is used to detect the organisms within clinical samples, using some form of complementary sequence and sometimes a signaling molecule. Signaling molecules are often some form of a fluorescent molecule to improve sensitivity.

DETECTION OF PATHOGENS WITHOUT AMPLIFICATION

The simplest application of molecular tools for the detection of infectious organisms is the use of a complementary nucleic acid sequence, termed a probe, which has been tagged with a fluorescent molecule. This probe is then added directly to a clinical sample, either a fluid or tissue section. Multiple probes, with different fluorescent tags, can be added to a single sample, allowing for the detection of several organisms in a single assay. This technique of hybridization of a probe to a target sequence in an organism was one of the first applied techniques in human clinical medicine but has not gained widespread use in feline medicine. This technique is still used routinely to monitor the viral load in patients infected with human immunodeficiency virus undergoing antiviral therapy. The feline therapeutic correlate, treatment of feline immunodeficiency virus (FIV), has not advanced to as finely tuned a protocol. Probe hybridization is rapid, user friendly, and simple to perform. This technique also removes the need for specialized culture conditions, but sensitivity of this technique is poor compared with other molecular techniques. Prior enrichment of the sample via microbiological culture improves sensitivity but increases the time needed for the assay and requires knowledge of the microbiological cultural demands of the organisms, eliminating many of the advantages of the technique for clinical application. This technique remains useful for the detection of slow-growing organisms, such as fungi and mycobacteria, in the presence of other more rapidly growing organisms in culture and for the rapid quantification of the organism load in a nonenriched clinical sample.

A more specialized application of probe hybridization is in situ hybridization. This technique uses the same theory as the simple probe hybridization but applies it to tissue samples, allowing the detection of the organisms of interest in association with inflammatory lesions or specific areas of tissue. This technique is useful in situations in which a large number of organisms can be detected, but the organisms may be part of a normal flora, such as those in the gastrointestinal tract. In situ hybridization allows the user to determine if certain bacterial species are associated with inflammation or are beyond the superficial layers of the gastrointestinal tract. Fluorescent molecules are the most common signaling mechanism used, and in this case, the method is abbreviated FISH (fluorescent in situ hybridization). The technology is as simple as a solution-based probe hybridization but requires skilled operators because nonspecific background staining can cause false-positive results.

DETECTION OF PATHOGENS WITH AMPLIFICATION: POLYMERASE CHAIN REACTION

The polymerase chain reaction (PCR) was first described in 1985[1] by Kary Mullis and colleagues, for which Mullis later received the Nobel Prize in Chemistry. This powerful tool uses the cyclic amplification of a strand of DNA using a proprietary enzyme to produce an exponential number of identical copies to a detectable level (**Fig. 1**A). The DNA is then analyzed, usually on a gel, to determine if it is of the predicted size for the reaction (see **Fig. 1**B). Application of this technique allows for the detection of minute numbers of organisms in a very small sample, an advantage in feline

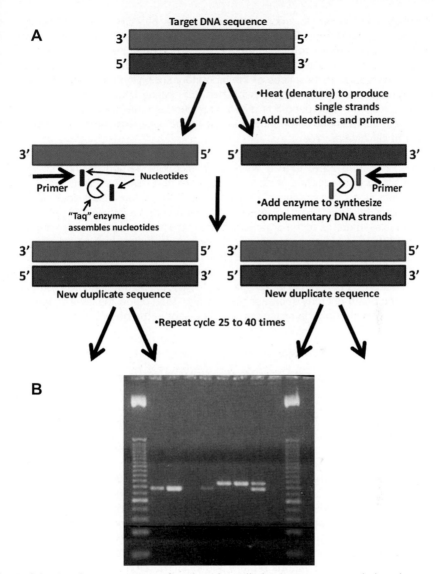

Fig. 1. (*A*) PCR. Short sequences of nucleotides called primers are annealed to the target DNA after the separation of the double strands. A proprietary enzyme is used to produce complementary strands of DNA during the synthesis step. Denaturation is repeated, and replication of the newly formed DNA strands, as well as the original target DNA, is repeated. (*B*) The DNA produced in the reaction (described in [*A*]) is then visualized using gel electro-phoresis. The size of the product is compared with a standard to confirm that the predicted product has been produced.

medicine given the size of patients. PCR is superior to probe hybridization techniques in sensitivity because of this amplification. Although the exponential amplification of the original target provides the greatest advantage of this technique, it is also the basis of the greatest downfall, contamination. Initially, PCR was restricted to highly specialized research and diagnostic laboratories. Commercially available kit-based technology now allows for more widespread use of PCR. This technology has decreased cost and improved availability but increases concerns regarding quality control. Strict adherence to good laboratory practice must be observed for credible results. This criterion raises a problem for clinicians because they cannot be aware of the actual laboratory practices of the laboratory supplying the assay. Therefore, it is recommended that if a recently published PCR assay is to be used clinically, the originating laboratory be used if at all possible because the laboratory personnel are familiar with the nuances of the individual assay and have experience with the largest number of clinical samples.

DNA of inactivated organisms injected into the bloodstream of laboratory animals has been detected more than a week after injection, demonstrating not only the high sensitivity of the technique but also the care that must be taken in interpreting results. Detection of an organism's nucleic acid in the bloodstream does not necessarily mean active infection or disease. The presence of nucleic acid simply indicates that the nucleic material of the organism exists in the host and not that the organism is alive, capable of replication, or actually causing clinical signs in the host. Correlation with clinical signs of a known syndrome associated with the organism and/or a response to therapy must be used in conjunction with the results of PCR. Finally, to prevent false-negative results, samples tested should be obtained before treatment because the treatment may decrease the organism load below the level of detection of even PCR, even though the organism is still present in the host.

PCR: VARIATIONS ON A THEME

Because of the structural differences between RNA and DNA, the enzyme used in PCR can only duplicate strands of DNA. However, many infectious agents are RNA viruses. Therefore, a preliminary step, reverse transcription (RT), to create a complementary strand of DNA from the target RNA must be performed. Amplification of the complementary DNA via PCR is then performed; this method is commonly known as RT-PCR.

The primers used in PCR can be designed to amplify the nucleic acids of only members of a certain genus, species, or even strain. The detection of suspected organisms is by far the most common use of PCR in veterinary medicine. When a single organism is targeted in an assay, the technique is termed a singleplex PCR. If multiple targets can be detected in a single assay, the technique is termed a multiplex assay. It is clearly most advantageous to investigate the presence of multiple organisms in a single assay. However, in the PCR assay, each target sequence competes with each other for the common building blocks that allow the reaction to proceed: the enzyme, nucleotide, and various buffers and ions. Therefore, multiplex reactions are frequently less sensitive than singleplex assays and require extensive optimization to be useful.

When no specific organism is identified as a likely cause of clinical signs, the use of broad-range or degenerate primers that amplify the DNA of the members of an entire genus or even kingdom can be used, targeting highly conserved regions of the nucleic acids. The most common application of PCR is for the rapid detection and identification of bacteria or fungi in clinical samples.[2,3] The PCR results can be available in as early as 2 hours and provides information on whether fungal or bacterial nucleic acids are present in the sample. Subsequent analysis of the PCR product may then be used to identify the infecting organism much more rapidly than traditional microbiological techniques and may be more sensitive for the detection of fastidious organisms. However, antimicrobial sensitivity is not available while using this technique; therefore, PCR is complementary to traditional culture techniques. However, the use of PCR for the detection of certain genes that encode for antimicrobial resistance is also starting to gain clinical use and may provide additional rapid information before antimicrobial sensitivity results are being available.[4]

The most recent application of PCR in clinical feline medicine has been real-time quantitative PCR (qPCR). Quantification by traditional endpoint PCR is difficult because after so many amplification cycles, most samples yield essentially the same amount of product because some limiting reagent would have been completely consumed before the final amplification cycles. In 1992, Higuchi and colleagues[5] reported a technique for monitoring the production of DNA during each amplification cycle so that the original quantity could be extrapolated by the identification of the log-arithmic amplification phase of each individual reaction. This technique uses fluores-cent dyes or probes that produce a signal after formation of the product (**Fig. 2**). During each amplification cycle, a detector records the amount of fluorescence in the sample. Gene expression is commonly measured using qPCR and has been used in many disease states in felines to evaluate host response to an infection.[6–12] Pathogen detection and load determination are some of the many applications of this technology. This assay has all the advantages of traditional endpoint PCR (sensi-tivity, specificity), offers a more rapid result, and has the ability to quantitate microbial DNA or RNA load. However, with these improvements additional concerns regarding quality control have been added. The fluorescent dyes and probes used to detect the PCR product allows for even more sensitive assays and susceptibility to contamina-tion leading to false-positive results. Accuracy of quantitation is reliant on the avail-ability of a reproducible high-quality standard curve. In an attempt to regulate this rapidly expanding field, minimum laboratory standards have been proposed.[13] Although these guidelines can be used to evaluate the quality of a published protocol, many diagnostic laboratories use proprietary reactions that are not subject to peer review. But because of this practice, the practitioner needs to request the evaluation data from the diagnostic laboratory to evaluate the clinical utility of the assay until it has been evaluated in a peer-reviewed journal.

MOLECULAR ASSAYS IN FELINE MEDICINE: CURRENT APPLICATIONS

The following is a review of assays that are currently commercially available in feline medicine for the diagnosis of infectious diseases. It is anticipated that many more applications will be developed in the upcoming years, and it is the responsibility of the clinician to maintain the knowledge of the current literature to apply these new assays in an appropriate manner. Molecular assays simply indicate the presence of a microbial DNA or RNA and not that of the disease. The ability of an assay to detect an organism is measured by its sensitivity and specificity: the frequency at which an assay can detect an organism (sensitivity) and not other organisms (specificity). The true measure of a test for disease diagnosis is the predictive value. Positive predictive value (PPV) is the measure of a test's ability to predict the presence of disease, and negative predictive value (NPV) is the ability of an assay to predict the absence of disease. However, most diagnostic laboratories can report only sensitivity and spec-ificity because they are easier to calculate, and hence the onus of remembering the predictive values of an assay for the syndrome being assessed is on the clinician.

Respiratory Agents

Feline calicivirus (FCV) infection is a common differential diagnosis in cats with clinical evidence of rhinitis and stomatitis. Less commonly, FCV infection is associated with conjunctivitis, polyarthritis, and lower airway disease in kittens. Virus isolation can

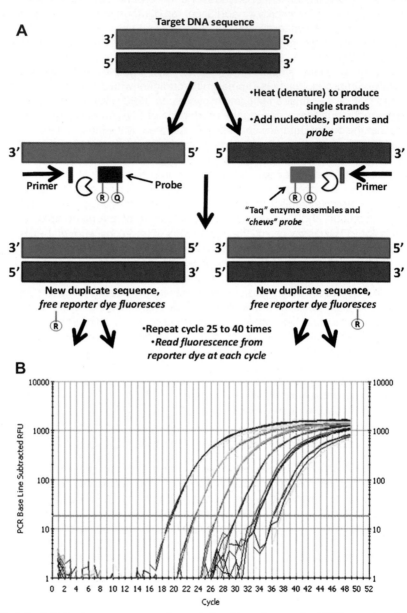

Fig. 2. (*A*) qPCR. In the most commonly used chemistry, the standard PCR assay is enhanced by using a fluorescent probe that fluoresces only after the removal of a quencher dye in close proximity to the reporter dye. The quencher dye is removed by the enzyme that synthesizes new strands of DNA as in traditional PCR. At each step, fluorescence is measured, allowing for the extrapolation of the amount of product present during each replication phase. (*B*) The change in fluorescence is then plotted against time (number of cycles), and a starting quantity can be calculated by the extrapolation of the signal produced during the exponential replication phase.

be used to document current infection but it takes at least several days for results to return. Because of widespread exposure and vaccination, the PPV of serologic tests is poor. RT-PCR assays can be used to amplify the RNA of FCV, and the results can be returned quickly. However, these assays also amplify vaccine strains of FCV. FCV RNA can be amplified from samples collected from normal carrier cats as well as from clinically ill cats, and so detection of FCV RNA has a poor PPV. For example, in one study, the presence of FCV RNA failed to correlate to the presence or absence of stomatitis in cats.[14] In addition, amplification of FCV RNA cannot be used to prove virulent systemic calicivirus infection. Results of FCV RT-PCR can also be false negative and so can have poor NPV.

Infection with feline herpesvirus 1 (FHV-1) is a common differential diagnosis in cats with clinical evidence of rhinitis, stomatitis, conjunctivitis, keratitis, and facial dermatitis. Because of widespread exposure and vaccination, the PPV of serologic tests is poor. FHV-1 can be documented by direct fluorescent staining of conjunctival scrapings, virus isolation, or PCR. FHV-1 DNA can be amplified from conjunctiva, nasal discharges, and pharynx of healthy cats, and so the PPV of conventional PCR assays is low.[15] Currently used PCR assays also detect vaccine strains of FHV-1, further lessening the PPV of the assays.[16] In one study, the presence of FHV-1 DNA failed to correlate to the presence or absence of stomatitis in cats.[14] In one study, results of qPCR may ultimately prove to correlate to the presence or absence of the disease but have failed to correlate to the presence of conjunctivitis.[17] The NPV of FHV-1 PCR assays is also in question because many cats that are likely to have FHV-1–associated disease show negative results. These results may relate to the clearance of FHV-1 DNA from tissues by a hypersensitivity reaction. Tissue biopsies have greater sensitivity than conjunctival swabs but do not necessarily have a greater predictive value. FHV-1 DNA can be amplified from the aqueous humor of some cats but whether this amplification indicates FHV-1–associated uveitis is unknown.

Mycoplasma spp, *Chlamydophila felis*, and *Bordetella bronchiseptica* are other common respiratory pathogens in cats. As for FHV-1 and FCV, PCR-positive test results cannot be used to distinguish a carrier from a clinically ill cat. In addition, PCR assays do not provide antimicrobial drug susceptibility testing, and so for cats with potential bordetellosis, culture and sensitivity is the optimal diagnostic technique, especially in case of an outbreak. *Toxoplasma gondii* DNA has been amplified from the airway washings of some cats with lower respiratory tract disease, and so PCR is an option for evaluation of samples from diseased animals from which the organism is not identified cytologically.

Gastrointestinal Agents

The detection of *Giardia* spp is generally made with the combination of fecal flotation techniques and wet-mount examination. Fecal antigen tests are also accurate, and there are several assays available for point-of-care use, including one labeled for veterinary use.[18] Fecal PCR assays often show false-negative results because of PCR inhibitors in stool, and so PCR should not be used as a screening procedure for this agent. However, *Giardia* spp PCR assays can be used to determine whether the infective species is a zoonotic assemblage, which is the primary indication for this technique. However, it now seems that assemblage determination should be performed on more than 1 gene for most accurate results.

Although *Cryptosporidium* spp infection is common, it is unusual to find *Cryptosporidium felis* oocysts using fecal flotation in cats. Acid-fast staining of a thin fecal smear is cumbersome and insensitive. Antigen assays titrated for use with human feces are inaccurate when used with cat feces. Thus, PCR may aid in the diagnosis of cryptosporidiosis in dogs and cats and has been shown to be more sensitive than immunofluorescence assays (IFAs) in cats.[19] *Cryptosporidium* spp PCR assays are indicated in IFA-negative cats with unexplained small bowel diarrhea and when the genotype of *Cryptosporidium* is to be determined. However, *Cryptosporidium felis* infection in cats is common, and so positive test results do not always prove that *Cryptosporidium felis* is the cause of the clinical disease. No drug is known to eliminate *Cryptosporidium* spp infections and small animal strains are not considered significant zoonotic agents; so PCR is not currently indicated in healthy animals. PCR assays are also available for the detection of DNA of *Tritrichomonas foetus*, *Salmonella* spp, *Campylobacter* spp, *Clostridium* spp, parvoviruses, and *T gondii*, and RT-PCR assay is available for coronaviruses. Trophozoites of *T foetus* can often be detected on wet-mount examination of fresh feces, which can be completed as an in-clinic test. The DNA of *T foetus* can be detected in healthy carrier cats, and so positive test results do not always prove illness from the organism.[20] In cases with suspected salmonellosis or campylobacteriosis, assessment should be done by culture rather than by PCR to determine the antimicrobial susceptibility patterns. In dogs, the PPV of *Clostridium* spp PCR assays on feces is low, and if the assay is used, it should be combined with enterotoxin assays. Information in cats is currently lacking. At present, there is noevidence that parvovirus PCR assays on feces is superior to currently available antigen assays and that currently used PCR assays for panleukopenia virus amplify vaccine strains. Oocysts of *T gondii* are shed only for about 7 to 10 days, and millions of oocysts are generally shed during this period, making the organism very easy to identify. Thus, PCR assays are usually not needed to diagnose this infection. Because virus isolation is not clinically practical, RT-PCR is used most frequently to detect coronavirus RNA in feces. However, positive test results do not differentiate feline infectious peritonitis (FIP)-inducing strains from enteric coronaviruses.

Blood-Borne Agents

Mycoplasma haemofelis (Mhf), Candidatus *Mycoplasma haemominutum* (Mhm), and Candidatus *Mycoplasma turicensis* (Mtc) can be found in cats. In at least 2 studies of experimentally infected cats, Mhf was found to be apparently more pathogenic than Mhm. It seems that Mtc has intermediate pathogenicity. Diagnosis is based on demonstration of the organism on the surface of erythrocytes on examination of a thin blood film or PCR assay. The number of organisms fluctuates, and so blood film examination results can be false negative up to 50% of the time. It may be difficult to find the agent cytologically, particularly in the chronic phase. Thus, PCR assays are the tests of choice because of their sensitivity.[21] Primers that can amplify the DNA of all the 3 hemoplasmas are available. qPCR assays can be used to monitor copy numbers during and after treatment but do not have greater sensitivity, specificity, or predictive value than conventional PCR assays.[22] PCR assays should be considered in the evaluation of cats with unexplained fever or anemia and that are cytologically negative for the hemoplasmas. In addition, the American College of Veterinary Internal Medicine recommends screening cats for hemoplasmas by PCR assays for their use as blood donors.[23] Many cats are carriers of the relatively nonpathogenic Candidatus Mhm, and so positive test results may not always correlate to the presence of the disease (poor PPV).

Cats can be infected by an *Ehrlichia canis*–like organism[24] and *Anaplasma phagocytophilum*.[25] Little is known about the other agents in these genera in regard to cats. Because the organisms are in different genera, serologic cross-reactivity is variable. Thus, although the clinical syndromes can be similar, there is neither a single serologic test to document infection nor a standardized serology for cats. In addition, some cats with *E canis* infection do not seroconvert, and so PCR assay is superior to serologic tests in cats. PCR assays can be designed to amplify the nucleic acid in each organism. Alternately, primers are available to amplify the entire nucleic acid of the organisms in a single reaction, and then sequencing can be used to determine the infective species.

Cats can be infected by *Rickettsia felis* and have been shown to have antibodies against *Rickettsia rickettsii*. Fever, headache, myalgia, and macular rash in humans have been attributed to *R felis* infection in several countries around the world. In a study, 92 pairs of cat blood and flea extracts from Alabama, Maryland, and Texas were assayed using PCR assays that amplify a region of the citrate synthase gene (*gltA*) and the outer membrane protein B gene (*ompB*). Of the 92 pairs, 62 (67.4%) flea extracts and none of the cat blood samples were positive for the presence of *R felis* DNA.[26] In another study, antibody prevalence rates of *R felis* and *R rickettsii* were shown to be 5.6% and 6.6%, respectively, in cats with fever, but neither DNA was amplified from blood.[27] These results proved that cats are sometimes exposed to these organisms, but further data are needed to determine the significance of disease associations. Whether *Rickettsia* spp PCR assays are indicated for use in cats at present is unknown.

Blood culture, PCR assay on blood, and serologic testing can be used to assess individual cats for *Bartonella* spp infection. Cats that are culture negative or PCR negative and antibody negative and cats that are culture negative or PCR negative and antibody positive are probably not a source of flea, cat, or human infection. However, bacteremia can be intermittent and false-negative culture or PCR results can occur, limiting the predictive value of a single battery of tests. Although serologic testing can be used to determine whether an individual cat has been exposed, both seropositive and seronegative cats can be bacteremic, limiting the diagnostic utility of serologic testing. Thus, testing healthy cats for *Bartonella* spp infection is not recommended at present.[28] Testing should be reserved for cats with suspected clinical bartonellosis. Because *Bartonella* spp infection is so common in healthy cats, even culture- or PCR-positive results do not prove clinical bartonellosis. For example, although DNA of *Bartonella* spp was detected in more number of cats with fever than in pair-matched cats without fever, the test results in healthy cats were still commonly positive.[29] A combination of serology and PCR is a rational approach to the evaluation of cats with suspected bartonellosis.

Cytauxzoon felis in clinically affected cats is usually easily identified on cytologic examination of blood smears or splenic aspirates. Serologic testing is not commercially available. PCR can be used to amplify the organism's DNA from the blood of cats that are cytologically negative for *Cytauxzoon felis*.[30]

Antibodies against FIV are detected in serum in clinical practice most frequently by enzyme-linked immunosorbent assay (ELISA). Comparisons between different tests have shown that the results of most assays are comparable.[31] Results of virus isolation or RT-PCR on blood are positive in some serologically negative cats. False-positive reactions can occur using ELISA; hence, positive results of ELISA in healthy or low-risk cats should be confirmed using Western blot immunoassay. Kittens can have detectable colostrum-derived antibodies for several months. Kittens younger than 6 months that are FIV seropositive should be tested every 60 days until the result is negative. If antibodies persist at 6 months of age, the kitten is likely infected. Virus isolation or RT-PCR on blood can also be performed to confirm infection. However, FIV is not present in the blood in high levels, and so false-negative test results are common. Thus, the assay is not very accurate for distinguishing a vaccinated cat from a naturally exposed cat.[32,33]

Most cats with feline leukemia virus infection are viremic, and so molecular diagnostic assays are not usually needed in clinical practice. However, newer sensitive qPCR assays have been used to accurately characterize the stages of infection[34,35] but these assays are not commonly available commercially.

RNA of both FIP virus and feline enteric coronavirus (FECV) can be amplified from the blood of cats, and so positive test results do not always correlate with the development of FIP. Amplification of the mRNA (messenger RNA) of the M gene by RT-PCR had mixed results in 2 studies performed to date. This amplification is a logical approach in theory and was found to have high specificity in the first report of this approach.[36] However, in a follow-up study with a larger number of cats, 13 of 26 apparently normal cats were positive for FECV mRNA in blood suggesting that the PPV of this assay for the diagnosis of FIP was low.[37] This assay is still available commercially; however, based on the published data, the assay does not seem to be anymore clinically useful than any other molecular assay for the diagnosis of FIP.

Ocular Agents

T gondii, Bartonella spp, FHV-1, and coronavirus are the organisms in which the DNA or RNA has been amplified most frequently from the aqueous humor of cats with endogenous uveitis. Although little is known about the predictive value of these assays when used with aqueous humor, the combination of molecular assays with local antibody production indices may aid in the diagnosis of some cases.

SUMMARY

As molecular tools become more widely available, the cost and availability of molecular assays become more accessible to feline practitioners. However, molecular diagnosis is a rapidly expanding field, and the sensitivity of these assays along with the often high frequency of detection in healthy animals makes interpretation of positive test results difficult. The clinician must remember that predictive value is a much more valuable tool for the assessment of the utility of a test result in a particular animal.

REFERENCES

1. Saiki RK, Scharf S, Faloona F, et al. Enzymatic amplification of beta-globin genomic sequences and restriction site analysis for diagnosis of sickle-cell anemia. Science 1985;230(4732):1350–4.
2. Schabereiter-Gurtner C, Nehr M, Apfalter P, et al. Evaluation of a protocol for molecular broad-range diagnosis of culture-negative bacterial infections in clinical routine diagnosis. J Appl Microbiol 2008;104(4):1228–37.
3. Lau A, Chen S, Sorrell T, et al. Development and clinical application of a panfungal PCR assay to detect and identify fungal DNA in tissue specimens. J Clin Microbiol 2007;45(2):380–5.
4. Mapes S, Rhodes DM, Wilson WD, et al. Comparison of five real-time PCR assays for detecting virulence genes in isolates of Escherichia coli from septicaemic neonatal foals. Vet Rec 2007;161(21):716–8.
5. Higuchi R, Dollinger G, Walsh PS, et al. Simultaneous amplification and detection of specific DNA sequences. Biotechnology (N Y) 1992;10(4):413–7.
6. Leutenegger CM, Boretti FS, Mislin CN, et al. Immunization of cats against feline immunodeficiency virus (FIV) infection by using minimalistic immunogenic defined gene expression vector vaccines expressing FIV gp140 alone or with feline interleukin-12 (IL-12), IL-16, or a CpG motif. J Virol 2000;74(22):10447–57.

7. Norris Reinero CR, Decile KC, Berghaus RD, et al. An experimental model of allergic asthma in cats sensitized to house dust mite or bermuda grass allergen. Int Arch Allergy Immunol 2004;135(2):117–31.

8. Veir JK, Lappin MR, Dow SW. Evaluation of a novel immunotherapy for treatment of chronic rhinitis in cats. J Feline Med Surg 2006;8(6):400–11.

9. Foley J, Hurley K, Pesavento PA, et al. Virulent systemic feline calicivirus infection: local cytokine modulation and contribution of viral mutants. J Feline Med Surg 2006;8(1):55–61.

10. Foley JE, Rand C, Leutenegger C. Inflammation and changes in cytokine levels in neurological feline infectious peritonitis. J Feline Med Surg 2003;5(6):313–22.

11. Gunn-Moore DA, Caney SM, Gruffydd-Jones TJ, et al. Antibody and cytokine responses in kittens during the development of feline infectious peritonitis (FIP). Vet Immunol Immunopathol 1998;65(2–4):221–42.

12. Harley R, Helps CR, Harbour DA, et al. Cytokine mRNA expression in lesions in cats with chronic gingivostomatitis. Clin Diagn Lab Immunol 1999;6(4):471–8.

13. Bustin SA, Benes V, Garson JA, et al. The MIQE guidelines: minimum information for publication of quantitative real-time PCR experiments. Clin Chem 2009;55(4):611–22.

14. Quimby JM, Elston T, Hawley J, et al. Evaluation of the association of Bartonella species, feline herpesvirus 1, feline calicivirus, feline leukemia virus and feline immunodeficiency virus with chronic feline gingivostomatitis. J Feline Med Surg 2008;10(1):66–72.

15. Veir JK, Ruch-Gallie R, Spindel ME, et al. Prevalence of selected infectious organisms and comparison of two anatomic sampling sites in shelter cats with upper respiratory tract disease. J Feline Med Surg 2008;10(6):551–7.

16. Maggs DJ, Clarke HE. Relative sensitivity of polymerase chain reaction assays used for detection of feline herpesvirus type 1 DNA in clinical samples and commercial vaccines. Am J Vet Res 2005;66(9):1550–5.

17. Low HC, Powell CC, Veir JK, et al. Prevalence of feline herpesvirus 1, Chlamydophila felis, and Mycoplasma spp DNA in conjunctival cells collected from cats with and without conjunctivitis. Am J Vet Res 2007;68(6):643–8.

18. Mekaru SR, Marks SL, Felley AJ, et al. Comparison of direct immunofluorescence, immunoassays, and fecal flotation for detection of Cryptosporidium spp. and Giardia spp. in naturally exposed cats in 4 Northern California animal shelters. J Vet Intern Med 2007;21(5):959–65.

19. Scorza AV, Brewer MM, Lappin MR. Polymerase chain reaction for the detection of Cryptosporidium spp. in cat feces. J Parasitol 2003;89(2):423–6.

20. Gookin JL, Stebbins ME, Hunt E, et al. Prevalence of and risk factors for feline Tritrichomonas foetus and giardia infection. J Clin Microbiol 2004;42(6):2707–10.

21. Jensen WA, Lappin MR, Kamkar S, et al. Use of a polymerase chain reaction assay to detect and differentiate two strains of Haemobartonella felis in naturally infected cats. Am J Vet Res 2001;62(4):604–8.

22. Tasker S, Helps CR, Day MJ, et al. Use of real-time PCR to detect and quantify Mycoplasma haemofelis and "Candidatus Mycoplasma haemominutum" DNA. J Clin Microbiol 2003;41(1):439–41.

23. Wardrop KJ, Reine N, Birkenheuer A, et al. Canine and feline blood donor screening for infectious disease. J Vet Intern Med 2005;19(1):135–42.

24. Breitschwerdt EB, Abrams-Ogg AC, Lappin MR, et al. Molecular evidence supporting Ehrlichia canis-like infection in cats. J Vet Intern Med 2002;16(6):642–9.

25. Lappin MR, Breitschwerdt EB, Jensen WA, et al. Molecular and serologic evidence of *Anaplasma phagocytophilum* infection in cats in North America. J Am Vet Med Assoc 2004;225(6):893–6, 879.

26. Hawley JR, Shaw SE, Lappin MR. Prevalence of *Rickettsia felis* DNA in the blood of cats and their fleas in the United States. J Feline Med Surg 2007;9(3):258–62.

27. Bayliss DB, Morris AK, Horta MC, et al. Prevalence of *Rickettsia* species antibodies and *Rickettsia* species DNA in the blood of cats with and without fever. J Feline Med Surg 2009;11(4):266–70.

28. Brunt J, Guptill L, Kordick DL, et al. American Association of Feline Practitioners 2006 Panel report on diagnosis, treatment, and prevention of *Bartonella* spp. infections. J Feline Med Surg 2006;8(4):213–26.

29. Lappin MR, Breitschwerdt E, Brewer M, et al. Prevalence of *Bartonella* species antibodies and *Bartonella* species DNA in the blood of cats with and without fever. J Feline Med Surg 2009;11(2):141–8.

30. Haber MD, Tucker MD, Marr HS, et al. The detection of *Cytauxzoon felis* in apparently healthy free-roaming cats in the USA. Vet Parasitol 2007;146(3–4):316–20.

31. Hartmann K, Griessmayr P, Schulz B, et al. Quality of different in-clinic test systems for feline immunodeficiency virus and feline leukaemia virus infection. J Feline Med Surg 2007;9(6):439–45.

32. Crawford PC, Slater MR, Levy JK. Accuracy of polymerase chain reaction assays for diagnosis of feline immunodeficiency virus infection in cats. J Am Vet Med Assoc 2005;226(9):1503–7.

33. Levy JK, Crawford PC, Kusuhara H, et al. Differentiation of feline immunodeficiency virus vaccination, infection, or vaccination and infection in cats. J Vet Intern Med 2008;22(2):330–4.

34. Cattori V, Hofmann-Lehmann R. Absolute quantitation of feline leukemia virus proviral DNA and viral RNA loads by TaqMan real-time PCR and RT-PCR. Methods Mol Biol 2008;42:973–87.

35. Torres AN, Mathiason CK, Hoover EA. Re-examination of feline leukemia virus: host relationships using real-time PCR. Virology 2005;332(1):272–83.

36. Simons FA, Vennema H, Rofina JE, et al. A mRNA PCR for the diagnosis of feline infectious peritonitis. J Virol Methods 2005;124(1–2):111–6.

37. Can-Sahna K, Ataseven VS, Pinar D, et al. The detection of feline coronaviruses in blood samples from cats by mRNA RT-PCR. J Feline Med Surg 2007;9(5):369–72.

Index

Note: Page numbers of article titles are in **boldface** type.

United States Postal Service

Statement of Ownership, Management, and Circulation
(All Periodicals Publications Except Requestor Publications)

1. Publication Title	2. Publication Number	3. Filing Date
Veterinary Clinics of North America: Small Animal Practice	0 0 3 - 1 5 0	9/15/10

4. Issue Frequency	5. Number of Issues Published Annually	6. Annual Subscription Price
Jan, Mar, May, Jul, Sep, Nov	6	$245.00

7. Complete Mailing Address of Known Office of Publication (Not printer) (Street, city, county, state, and ZIP+4®)

Elsevier Inc.
360 Park Avenue South
New York, NY 10010-1710

Contact Person
Stephen Bushing
Telephone (Include area code)
215-239-3688

8. Complete Mailing Address of Headquarters or General Business Office of Publisher (Not printer)

Elsevier Inc., 360 Park Avenue South, New York, NY 10010-1710

9. Full Names and Complete Mailing Addresses of Publisher, Editor, and Managing Editor (Do not leave blank)

Publisher (Name and complete mailing address)

Kim Murphy, Elsevier, Inc., 1600 John F. Kennedy Blvd. Suite 1800, Philadelphia, PA 19103-2899

Editor (Name and complete mailing address)

John Vassallo, Elsevier, Inc., 1600 John F. Kennedy Blvd. Suite 1800, Philadelphia, PA 19103-2899

Managing Editor (Name and complete mailing address)

Catherine Bewick, Elsevier, Inc., 1600 John F. Kennedy Blvd. Suite 1800, Philadelphia, PA 19103-2899

10. Owner (Do not leave blank. If the publication is owned by a corporation, give the name and address of the corporation immediately followed by the names and addresses of all stockholders owning or holding 1 percent or more of the total amount of stock. If not owned by a corporation, give the names and addresses of the individual owners. If owned by a partnership or other unincorporated firm, give its name and address as well as those of each individual owner. If the publication is published by a nonprofit organization, give its name and address.)

Full Name	Complete Mailing Address
Wholly owned subsidiary of	4520 East-West Highway
Reed/Elsevier, US holdings	Bethesda, MD 20814

11. Known Bondholders, Mortgagees, and Other Security Holders Owning or Holding 1 Percent or More of Total Amount of Bonds, Mortgages, or Other Securities. If none, check box ☑ None

Full Name	Complete Mailing Address
N/A	

12. Tax Status (For completion by nonprofit organizations authorized to mail at nonprofit rates) (Check one)
The purpose, function, and nonprofit status of this organization and the exempt status for federal income tax purposes:
☐ Has Not Changed During Preceding 12 Months
☐ Has Changed During Preceding 12 Months (Publisher must submit explanation of change with this statement)

PS Form 3526, September 2007 (Page 1 of 3 (Instructions Page 3)) PSN 7530-01-000-9931 **PRIVACY NOTICE:** See our Privacy policy in www.usps.com

13. Publication Title	14. Issue Date for Circulation Data Below
Veterinary Clinics of North America: Small Animal Practice	September 2010

15. Extent and Nature of Circulation			Average No. Copies Each Issue During Preceding 12 Months	No. Copies of Single Issue Published Nearest to Filing Date
a. Total Number of Copies (Net press run)			2779	2513
b. Paid Circulation (By Mail and Outside the Mail)	(1)	Mailed Outside-County Paid Subscriptions Stated on PS Form 3541. (Include paid distribution above nominal rate, advertiser's proof copies, and exchange copies)	1573	1478
	(2)	Mailed In-County Paid Subscriptions Stated on PS Form 3541 (Include paid distribution above nominal rate, advertiser's proof copies, and exchange copies)		
	(3)	Paid Distribution Outside the Mails Including Sales Through Dealers and Carriers, Street Vendors, Counter Sales, and Other Paid Distribution Outside USPS®	406	408
	(4)	Paid Distribution by Other Classes Mailed Through the USPS (e.g. First-Class Mail®)		
c. Total Paid Distribution (Sum of 15b (1), (2), (3), and (4))			1979	1886
d. Free or Nominal Rate Distribution (By Mail and Outside the Mail)	(1)	Free or Nominal Rate Outside-County Copies Included on PS Form 3541	102	94
	(2)	Free or Nominal Rate In-County Copies Included on PS Form 3541		
	(3)	Free or Nominal Rate Copies Mailed at Other Classes Through the USPS (e.g. First-Class Mail)		
	(4)	Free or Nominal Rate Distribution Outside the Mail (Carriers or other means)		
e. Total Free or Nominal Rate Distribution (Sum of 15d (1), (2), (3) and (4))			102	94
f. Total Distribution (Sum of 15c and 15e)			2081	1980
g. Copies not Distributed (See instructions to publishers #4 (page #3))			698	533
h. Total (Sum of 15f and g)			2779	2513
i. Percent Paid (15c divided by 15f times 100)			95.10%	95.25%

16. Publication of Statement of Ownership

If the publication is a general publication, publication of this statement is required. Will be printed ☑ Publication not required
in the November 2010 issue of this publication.

17. Signature and Title of Editor, Publisher, Business Manager, or Owner

Stephen R. Bushing Date

Stephen R. Bushing Fulfillment/Inventory Specialist September 15, 2010

I certify that all information furnished on this form is true and complete. I understand that anyone who furnishes false or misleading information on this form or who omits material or information requested on the form may be subject to criminal sanctions (including fines and imprisonment) and/or civil sanctions (including civil penalties).

PS Form 3526, September 2007 (Page 2 of 3)

Moving?

Make sure your subscription moves with you!

To notify us of your new address, find your **Clinics Account Number** (located on your mailing label above your name), and contact customer service at:

Email: journalscustomerservice-usa@elsevier.com

800-654-2452 (subscribers in the U.S. & Canada)
314-447-8871 (subscribers outside of the U.S. & Canada)

Fax number: 314-447-8029

Elsevier Health Sciences Division
Subscription Customer Service
3251 Riverport Lane
Maryland Heights, MO 63043

*To ensure uninterrupted delivery of your subscription,
please notify us at least 4 weeks in advance of move.